Laughter Mastery

Jeffrey Briar

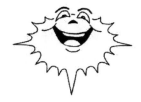

Laughter

Mastery

For Laughter Yoga
Trainings
and Advanced Education

Jeffrey Briar

Laughter Mastery

For Laughter Yoga Trainings and Advanced Education

ISBN-13: **978-1979714464**

ISBN-10: **1979714460**

Creative Arts Press
790 Manzanita Drive
Laguna Beach, California USA 92651
(949) 376-1939
www.LYInstitute.org
Email: Info@LYInstitute.org

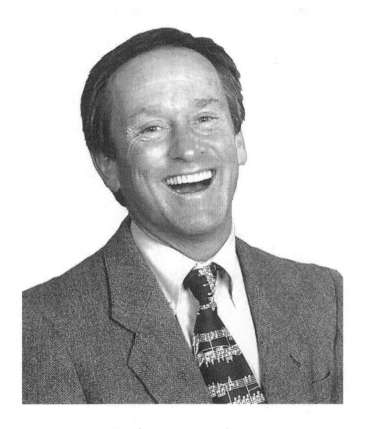

By the same author:

The Laughter Yoga Book
Laughter Exercises: The Great Big Anthology
Laughter Revolutionaries: Making the World Safe for Hilarity
Moving Experiences: A Manual for Awakening
Froigen deebled Craggle-Zorp! (The All-Gibberish Storybook)
DVD: *The Laughter Club in Real Time*
DVD: *Gibberish Sets You Free*
DVD: *Gibberish Kit* (with Dr. Madan Kataria)

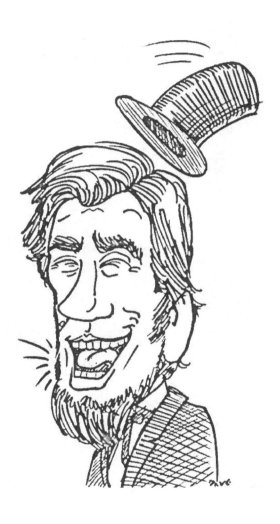

-- Art by David Fleischmann

Table of Contents

A definition of "happiness" according to Doctors Earl Henslin (*This Is Your Brain on Joy*) and Lee Berk, two of the world's most prominent psychoneuroimmunologists:

"Happiness is
dopaminergic
upregulation
in the
nucleus accumbens
of the brain."

PREFACE

Welcome to *Laughter Mastery*, a collection of learning aids compiled during twelve years of educational programs delivered by the author, a senior trainer in the Laughter Yoga technique.

The fundamental practice consists of laughing voluntarily, without needing jokes nor comedy. Laughter is practiced as a *Participatory* Activity: we simply "do it", like attending an enjoyable exercise class. This is not laughter as a Spectator Sport, like going to a ballgame (or a comedy nightclub) where we passively witness others doing the real work, and we laugh as a reaction to their efforts - if/when we find them sufficiently amusing. A Laughter Yoga session is filled with laughter performed *pro-actively*, as a choice; we don't wait for something amusing to happen to cause us to laugh as a *re-action*. "Laughter is too important to leave to chance."

This book is designed to support the learning and dissemination of the delightful and empowering Laughter Yoga technique, with its vision of health, happiness, and world peace through people laughing together. The contents range from simple statements of basic practices to profound developments of the principles of applied therapeutic laughter.

The why, how, and benefits of deliberate laughing will be found in the pages following. For an abundance of profusely illustrated hands-on techniques, see the publication *Laughter Exercises: The Great Big Anthology* by the same author.

Our world has changed substantially during the twelve years when these writings were assembled. In the early days, Laughter Yoga practitioners celebrated with glee when *anything* related to laughter-for-health appeared in the news, anywhere on earth. Now, hardly a day goes by without an article appearing somewhere on the planet, praising laughter for its diverse benefits.

The author's heartfelt thanks and gratitude go out to Doctor Madan Kataria and his lovely wife Madhuri, the sources and founders of this extraordinary work whereby everyone can share friendship, fun, and caring relationships, through voluntary laughter without the need of comedy – without, in fact, the need for shared language nor common cultures. Everybody loves to laugh. Blessings on Madan and Madhuri for designing this method whereby everyone on earth can share the heartfelt, happiness-inducing activity of laughing together as one joyful family.

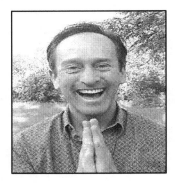

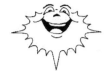 **LAUGHTER YOGA**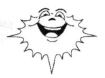

Why laugh?

In the 1960s journalist Norman Cousins cured himself of a painful disease (which had been diagnosed as terminal) by checking into a hotel room and watching a steady supply of funny movies and TV shows. His acclaimed book *Anatomy of an Illness* told the tale of his recovery and led to extensive medical research.

Benefits of Laughter may include:
* Relieves stress: reduces adrenaline and cortisol)
* Reduces anxiety, fear, depression; raises serotonin levels
* Relieves pain: produces endorphins, the body's natural pain-killing "feel-good" hormones - or at least has an endorphin-like effect; generates the natural Chemistry of Happiness
* Enhances the immune system: increases lymphocytes, moves the lymph, boosts natural anti-viral and anti-cancer cell activity)
* Improves respiratory and cardiovascular systems: dilates blood vessels, balances blood pressure; increases lung capacity, raises oxygen levels in the blood
* Improves sleep patterns
* Benefits digestion and elimination systems (sometimes described as "internal jogging")
* Encourages relaxation
* Boosts self-confidence, promotes compassion, deepens creativity

It is said that children may laugh hundreds of times each day, yet most adults are lucky if we laugh fifteen times - in a *good* day. (Can you remember the last time you laughed 100 times in one day? At a Laughter Yoga session you can anticipate laughing 100 times in ½ of one *hour!*) When we practice intentional laughter not only do we reduce our general stress level, we also actually develop our sense of humor. We are more likely to find things amusing and are able to see the lighter, brighter side of life.

"Laughter does not solve your problems, but it can help dissolve your problems." -- Dr. Kataria

When we laugh, even for no reason, the damaging effects of stress are neutralized and we return to a state of balance and peace.

With the practice Laughter Yoga, *you need never be "stressed out" again*.

What is "Laughter Yoga"?

Laughter Yoga is the brainchild of Doctor Madan Kataria, a physician from Bombay India, trained in Western medicine; and his wife Madhuri, a yoga teacher. In 1995 Dr. Kataria was studying the published research in order to write an article entitled "Laughter: The Best Medicine." He resolved to experience for himself the benefits of a consistent daily laughter practice. Kataria convinced a handful of people in a park in Bombay, who regularly went there to do walking as exercise, to add laughter practice for a while. After two weeks of using jokes and funny stories as a stimulus to laugh the members grew tired of hearing the same old lines, and some jokes were found offensive or simply not amusing. Dr. Kataria promised to come up with a way to laugh without resorting to jokes or humor; a method whereby people could

laugh at will, as a form of exercise to improve one's health
and sense of well-being.

"Laughter is too important to be dependent on jokes." --
-- Dr. Kataria

Some of the earliest laughter exercises were adaptations of
Yoga postures and breathing techniques: Lion, Mountain,
Salutation to the Sun, Breath of Fire, etc. Dr. Kataria
enhanced these practices by replacing yoga's typically quiet
exhalations with unconditional laughter. To everyone's
delight it was soon discovered that any forced laughter
rapidly became genuine heartfelt laughter when done in the
company of other mirth-minded people. Even if the laughter
started out "fake" it soon became real.

"As far as your health is concerned,
laughing from having fun
is just as good as laughing *at* something funny."
-- Jeffrey Briar

Research has shown that whether laughter is voluntary
(self-generated) or reactive (externally triggered), the body
produces the physiological benefits of hearty hilarity.

There are now thousands of Laughter Clubs throughout
the world - more than 5,000 in India alone - and the number
is growing rapidly.

A typical laughter session would include: easy stretches,
breathing practices, and an assortment of intentional laughter
techniques. These are simple to follow and very pleasant to
perform. The individual can choose their level of
participation, from gentle to vigorous; the experience is

suitable for all ages and all levels of ability. In addition to the numerous health benefits, laughter buddies tend to form caring, supportive friendships.

If it's not about stretching, why use the word "Yoga"?

Laughter Yoga is based in breathing techniques (*Pranayama*) from traditional Yoga, except laughter is performed in place of the typically silent exhalation.

On a deeper level, the Sanskrit word *Yoga* translates as "union" or "yoke". It describes a philosophical path towards the individual's union with their own true nature. There are many styles or paths of Yoga, accommodating the differing dispositions of different people. There are paths focused on actions, prayer, study, or awakening physical/spiritual energies.

The most well-known style of Yoga is *Ha-tha* (Sanskrit words meaning "sun-moon"), which is concerned with balancing energies and is enacted by the famous Yoga postures or *asanas* which stretch the physical body in various balanced ways.

Doctor Kataria developed, and continues to develop, a path he has named Hasya Yoga (*hasya* is the Sanskrit word for laughter). Through Laughter Yoga practices, the individual: deepens their breathing, improves their physical health, releases negative thoughts/emotions, and gets in touch with their spiritual nature. This leads effortlessly to attitudes of compassion, forgiveness, kindness, and actively seeking the happiness of others.

In this way, Laughter Yoga truly is a yogic path. It does not require the physical dexterity and stretching of *Hatha Yoga*; nonetheless, Laughter Yoga practice does have numerous physical benefits, as well as bringing tranquility, joy and love to the mind and soul; the same spiritual benefits desired by all paths of Yoga.

The ultimate mission of Laughter Yoga is World Peace through Laughter.
(No kidding.)

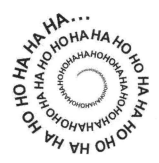

"Ho ho ha ha Spiral" from and © Laughter Yoga International

Written by and © Jeffrey Briar
CLYT (Certified Laughter Yoga Teacher) and
Master Trainer for Laughter Yoga University

Permission to reprint the above article (pps. 9-13 only) is granted providing that writing credit is given to author, along with a link to either
A.) The website **www.LYInstitute.org**
or
B.) Email address **JBriar@LYInstitute.org**

Laughter Yoga Basics

(The Cheat Sheet)

WHAT IS A LAUGHTER CLUB?

"A group of p_____ who gather together

to practice l_____

as a form of e_____ to improve their health.

And, they have a lot of f_____ doing it."

("They reconnect with a c_____ sense
 of playfulness.")

KEY CONCEPT (Voluntary Laughter) :

You don't need to feel g_____,

have any r_____,

or even have a sense of h_____

in order to l_____.

If you laugh, even for no reason, soon you do feel
good, and the laughing improves your sense of
humor.

WHY IS IT CALLED "LAUGHTER YOGA"?

For thousands of years, traditional Hatha Yoga has
shown that breathing practices can influence
the body, mind and emotions.

Laughter Yoga combines laughter exercises with
Yoga breathing practices ("Pranayama") to
create a *joyful* Body-Mind experience.

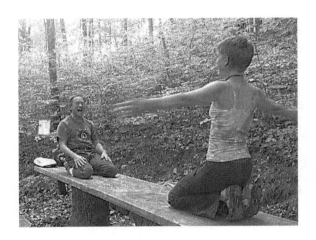

What Is Laughter Yoga
(in Five Points)

The "Under-One-Minute" Explanation

1. Laughter Yoga is a new technique whereby anyone can laugh without the need of jokes, comedy, or even having a sense of humor.

   You can start laughing even if you are feeling sad, angry, depressed - *any* emotion. So long as you are willing to laugh, you can do so.

2. Laughter Yoga is based in the scientifically demonstrated principle that even if laughter is voluntary, as long as it is performed with willingness, the Body does not make a distinction. Your Mind may think that the laughter is "pretend" but your Body will create the same physiological benefits as if the laughter was "real".

3. The laughter is performed as a form of Group Exercise. When we see others laughing, in an environment of playfulness and with good eye contact the laughter becomes contagious and soon it *does* become "real".

4. It is called Laughter "Yoga" because it combines Laughter Exercises with Yogic deep breathing practices known as *Pranayama*. This brings more oxygen to the body and brain, so we feel more healthy and energetic.

5. Laughter Yoga was developed by a medical doctor, Madan Kataria, in collaboration with his lovely wife Madhuri, a yoga teacher. They began with a group of five people in a park in Mumbai, India in 1995. Today there are thousands of laughter clubs all over the world.

-- Dr. Madan Kataria,
edited and with additions by Jeffrey Briar

Three Reasons: Why Do Laughter Yoga; Why Go to a Laughter Club (Three "Ds")

A person says: "I laugh throughout the day. I tell jokes at
work and watch comedy TV shows at night. Isn't that
enough? Why should I go to a Laughter Class?"

Response:

In order to get the proven health benefits of laughter, there are
a few requirements.

1.   Duration

We need to laugh continuously for 10 to 15 minutes. Typical
laughter occurs for only a few moments here and there, but
this is not adequate to have significant physiological effects.
15 minutes of hearty laughter changes us into a biochemically
transformed person – someone who has just had a great time
laughing.

2.   Depth

The healthiest laughter must be deep, engaging the thoracic
diaphragm and abdominal muscles. Loud, deep laughter from
the belly may not be acceptable in many social circumstances
but at a Laughter Club hearty belly laughter is encouraged.

3.   Dependability

Typical laughter depends on conditions - we cannot count on
it. But at a Laughter Club we do laughter deliberately, as a
choice; we do not leave our laughter to chance. You can rely
on it: at a Laughter Club you will laugh abundantly, so long
as you are willing, because you choose to do so.

How to Lead a Laughter Exercise

The 3-D Technique (also known as **"Say, Show, 'Go!'"**)

All laughter exercise sessions begin with the advice that
   students can participate at whatever energy level they wish.
   They are welcome to modify any practice to suit their
   personal comfort level, or refrain from performing any
   activity which they think might cause them discomfort.

The Three "D's": Declare, Demonstrate, and "Cue to *Do*"
("Say, Show, 'Go!'")

**"Before starting any exercise, give its name, tell how to do it and
demonstrate."** (Kataria; 2017 Leader Manual, p. 52)

Step 1: *Declare* (Denote/De-name). **SAY** Name the exercise.

Example: "The next exercise is called Penguin Laughter."

Step 2: *Demonstrate.* **SHOW** Display how to perform the
   exercise, simultaneously verbalizing the instruction.

Example: "Start with your feet turned out [*place your feet in
   this position*], arms straight down by your sides, hands
   flexed, palms facing the floor. Walk around like a penguin
   [*do a stiff-legged walk, upward-flexed hands swinging away from
   and then towards the legs*]. Play with the other penguins,
   laughing all the while [*make eye contact with other participants
   while laughing, lean towards them in greeting*]."

Step 3: *Do.* (Give the "Cue to Do") **"GO!"** First: stop the
   demonstration. Then: give a clear command to start: the
   "Cue to Do". Do this with a sense of building up tension
   such that everyone will release into laughing together, all at
   the same time, the moment you give them the cue to do so.

Example: "Okay, 'feet turned out? Ready – set: *Start!*" (immediately burst into laughter). Or: "Penguins, are you ready? *Take off!*" Or: "Here we go: 1, 2, 3… W*addle!*"

[The main proponents of voluntary laughter are consistent in their direction to give a clear command for everyone to begin laughing at once. Kataria: **"The most important skill of a leader is to give commands for participants to start the exercise together and laugh at the same time."** (2017 Leader Manual, p. 51). Steve Wilson: **"Leader uses a count-down to get everyone laughing at the same time."** (2006 Manual, p. 26)]

Allow the exercise to run for at least fifteen seconds (thirty to forty-five seconds is preferred). Some enthusiastic groups may continue for an entire minute or longer. Tune in to your team. Allow for space wherein participants can go beyond their initial effort. Give them time to explore nuances and get in touch with their creative side.

Conclude the exercise by calling out words of praise (e.g.: "Great job, everyone!" or "That was fantastic!"; see Encouraging Words, pp. 43-46) or doing the "Ho, ho, ha-ha-ha" (p. 35) or "Very good, very good, Yay!" practice (p. 36).

Dozens of examples of laughter exercises being led and performed are available for viewing on YouTube. Visit the accounts under "JoyfulGent" and "Jeffrey Briar", or search under "laughter exercise briar."

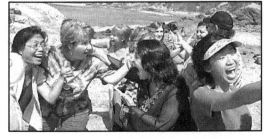

Cellphone Laughter

Warming Up the Voice

by **Kathryn Burns** with Jeffrey Briar

The voice is an essential element for participating in and
leading laughter exercises. Laughter is, after all, a
wonderful "vocalization"! When used correctly, your vocal
instrument will become stronger, richer, and more
powerful.

Like any muscle, the vocal chords respond well to: warming
up; **exercise which starts gently within a small range and
gradually expands that range**; and consistently correct
usage. Conversely, if strained or forced too quickly, the
vocal chords can become sore or even injured.

Laughter is a beautiful gift and **does not harm the voice**.
Natural laughter comes from deep in our belly, with full
involvement of the diaphragm. The throat and vocal chords
are loose and energized, expressive yet calm. If you feel
strain, laugh with an **open throat** from **deep down**
("Brooklyn Cab Driver") instead of up high and nasal
(whiny "Jerry Lewis").

We urge you to commit to a vocal warm up before leading,
and to incorporate vocal exercises as part of the total
experience of healthy, unconditional shared laughter.
Enjoy!

Elements of Healthy Vocal Hygiene

Relaxed, stretched, nourished and energized; involving the full body

Abdominal breathing (felt into the deep belly)

Throat relaxed

Projection (volume) supported by breath

Rich vocal resonance

Articulation – produce clear sounds (consonants distinct from vowels)

Expressive pitch variety

Constant hydration (swallow often, and drink water)

An excellent way to begin your warm up is in a hot steamy bath or shower. **Sing in the shower** – it's fun!

*Make humming sounds with an open throat (like yawing with the lips open). This bathes the vocal chords and gently awakens them.

* Make **nasal sounds**. These start to stretch the vocalizing muscles while protecting the throat.

* The **tongue:** alternately roll, extend, bend, and flutter.

* Open and close the **jaw**, circle it around (while making yawning, growling or singing sounds).
* Speak **gibberish**.
* Start by making a **pitch** and **raise it up and down** a small amount. Gradually, over several minutes' time, increase the range, higher and lower, as you continue. Do similarly with **volume**: Start at a moderate level; then make the sounds louder, then quieter. Keep varying the volume.
* **Sing**, using both traditional vocal warm-ups ("La la la LA la la la; li li li LI li li li, etc.) and "la la la" syllables while singing songs you know ("Twinkle Twinkle," any national anthem, "Happy Birthday," etc.). Also sing in gibberish. (Note: Unless you are doing an organized song (which is fine), discourage singing in "real" words, as the use of words can distract the other vocalizers.)
* Relax. * Breathe. * ...and of course: *Laugh!*

-> **Laughter Club Session Suggested Outline** <- p.1

Welcome: "No New Pain" - can always modify, or sit out

"Refrain from Talking" – once the laughter has begun, refrain from talking until the end of the session

Warm-Up stretches; add vocalization

Breathing Exercises

Breathing Exercises with laughter on outbreath

Laughter Exercises (15-20 minutes)

  *Greeting (Namaste); "Ho, ho, ha-ha-ha"

  *2 Exercises (H,H, h-h-h); Easy stretch/breathing

  *1 Exercise; "Very good, very good, yay!"

CONTINUES...

-> Laughter Club Session Outline <- p.2

*1 Exercise; Easy stretch/breathing

* 6 to 8 more exercises, interspersed with

(H,H, h-h-h), (VG, VG, Y!), and other easy

stretches/breathing exercises

Positive Affirmations

Laughter Meditation

Guided Relaxation

Wish for Peace; Announcements

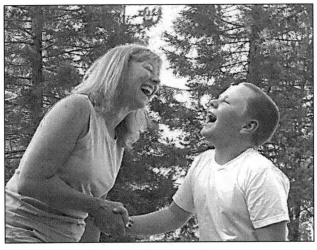

Handshake Laughter

Dr. Kataria's Original Foundation Exercises
(updates from 2015 begin on p. 38)

All Laughter Exercises are done "...while laughing."

Greeting Laughter

1. Indian Greeting, or Namaste Place the palms of the hands together in front of your heart. Bow slightly, keeping eye contact.

2. Western Greeting, or Handshake Shake hands and laugh robustly.

3. Double Handshake Laughter One person crosses hands, shakes two hands at a time with the other: up and down, in and out, side to side, etc.

4. Electric Shock Laughter Reach as if to shake hands -- imagine an electrostatic shock from the other person's hand. Fun surprise!

Laughter Exercises

Aloha Laughter Inhaling, raise both arms up; say "Alo---" for a long breath; at the very end of the breath, come down with a firm "Ha-a-a!" and continue to laugh deeply.

American Laughter Slap the thighs (like a cowboy from the Old West), one or both; place fists on hips. Big, broad, roaring laughs: "Yee-haw" and "Haw haw!"

Appreciation Laughter The tip of the index finger is joined to the tip of the thumb to make a small circle; or use a "thumbs-up" gesture. Can also applaud briefly; throw kisses; "give me high-five", etc.

Argument Laughter (aka "Naughty-Naughty") Pretend to "argue" by pointing and waggling index fingers at each other. Follow (and combine) with Forgiveness Laughter.

Bird Laughter Extend arms like a bird; flap "wings", take off, drift and fly (all different directions). *Variations*: *"Chicken Laughter"* If small space: bend elbows, fingertips on shoulders: flap and move around like chickens. *"Penguin Laughter"* Feet turned out, arms by sides, palms facing the ground; waddle around like penguins.

Calcutta Laughter With hands in front: two short sharp repetitions of "Ho, Ho" with hands pushing forward on each exhalation; followed by two short repetitions of "Ha, Ha" with hands facing down and pushing sharply downwards on each exhalation. Include a slight bounce in the knees.

Cellphone Laughter Hold an imaginary cell phone; it "rings," put it to your ear; laugh at what you hear. Move around and share with others (they laugh at yours, you laugh at theirs).

Creative Laughter One at a time, each person does spontaneous and playful: **1. Sounds, 2. Faces/Grimaces,**

and 3. Actions/Gestures, for a minute, while the others observe and react playfully. *Variations:* **1.** *"Follow the Leader"* Each person does some movement/laughter exercise for 10 to 60 seconds, the others copying them at the same time. **2.** One person holds an object (stick, scarf, ball, etc.) and does playful creative movements with it, while everyone laughs along. After a few seconds, pass the object to the next person. Everyone gets a turn.

Credit Card Bill Laughter In two hands hold an imaginary bill; open the hands (palms towards you) and laugh at what you see; share with others.

Crying Laughter Cry while sliding down to a crouch; then happily laugh your way up.

Elevator Laughter Stand close together in a group, laughing nervously as the elevator jiggles, doors open and close, bouncing around.

Forgiveness Laughter Offer forgiveness, arms apart and palms open: forgive yourself, forgive others.

Gradient Laughter and Silent Gradient Laughter Start with a smile, let it grow to a giggle; start gentle, and then allow to build (vigor and volume) slowly until roaring. Just allow it to be – no need to force it.

Guru Laughter Place one hand atop the head, "I learn from my mistakes, Hahahahaha!" Place the other hand atop the head: "I learn from others' mistakes, Hahahahaha!" Walk around making eye contact, admitting your humility.

Hot Sand Laughter Walking on very hot sand. Yeow!- ha-ha-ha-ha.

Hot Soup Laughter Stick out the tongue, shake hands up and down at wrists as if you have just had very hot, spicy soup; wave heat off the tongue.

Hugging Laughter (aka "Heart to Heart" or "Intimacy Laughter") Laugh as you gently hug one another, feel each other's laughter. (Note: Some may wish to only hold hands, or even hug the air around each other, without touching. Be sensitive to the other person's level of comfort.)

Jackpot Laughter (follows "No Money Laughter") Produce winning lottery ticket (or gold nugget), raise arms in celebration: we're rich!

Just Laughing (aka "We're Laughing for No Reason") A passerby has just asked, "Why are you all laughing?" Palms up, elbows bent, shoulders shrug, "We're just... laughing, for no reason!"

Laugh at Yourself Point finger at your heart area (may use both hands) – with a small movement, "It's okay to laugh at myself, I don't need to be perfect". Can point to head, belly, etc.

Laughter Center   Point finger to head; seek, find, and indicate the Brain's "Laughter Center" (could be anywhere: temple, crown, occipital ridge in back).   *Variation: "Find the Laugh"* – point to various body parts, questioning "Where is it?"; every 3rd place pointed to is where the Laughter is located; show to others.

Laughter Cream (aka "Giggle Cream" and "Laughter Lotion")   Squeeze tube into hand (or scoop out of a jar), then apply (to self, and to others).

Laughter Orchestra   People group into (laughter) instrument sections, conductor directs (laugh when pointed at; stop when the "Stop" gesture is done; get louder, softer, etc.).

Lion Laughter   Stick tongue way out and down towards the chin, big smile on cheeks; eyebrows lift high, eyes open wide; hands like a lion's paws, roar laughter from belly.

Mental Floss Laughter   Wrap floss around hands; "clean-out" the brain, tongue, between and around any and all body parts.

Milk Curd Laughter (aka "Churning Butter")   There's a churning stick in a barrel; lift the stick up & down; or (as if a rope attached) in back-&-forth movements, with repetitive laugh-sounds (as in "Tak-Choom" sounds).

Milkshake Laughter   Hold two imaginary glasses of milk. Pour one into the other, saying, "Aeee...", pour the second

into the first, saying (a little higher) "Aeeee ..."; then
pretend to drink: "Aee-ah-ha-ha-ha-ha!". *Variations*: 1.
After mixing, you start to drink ; it tastes funny, so you a.
toss it behind your back; or b. pour onto the ground in front
of you. 2. Share with others, by pouring down their backs,
in their hair, etc. – a pleasant and delightful gift!

Motorbike Laughter & Variations Start the engine in 3 laughs,
then drive around in your laugh-powered bike.

No Money Laughter (aka "Empty Pockets") (can precede
"Jackpot Laughter") Show empty pockets, laugh with
palms up.

One Meter Laughter As if measuring a length of cloth, start
with arms raised up to one side, the hands close together.
Move one arm along front of body, as if measuring: 1) to the
other arm's elbow, saying "Ae"; 2) to the same arm's
shoulder joint, saying (a little higher) "Ae"; then 3) arms
wide apart, head slightly back: "Aee-ah-ha-ha-ha-ha!"
laugh heartily, celebrating your having succeeded in
measuring a meter.

(One Meter Variant:) *One Centimeter Laughter* Measure just
from thumb tip to thumb joint; it's over so fast!

Royal Laughter Hand gently open, wave like the Queen of
England (rotating the forearm at the elbow joint).

Shy Laughter Hands in front of face, giggling; peek out
sometimes, laugh; then cover the face again.

Silent Laughter   As if someone is sleeping in the adjoining room, laugh very quietly so as to not wake them up. Can gently "Shush!" each other.

Touch the Sky (aka "Vowel Sounds," "Vowel Movement") Wide circle holding hands. Move forward, saying each vowel sound, raising hands and bursting into laughter as arrive in the center. First time: A (ay); then E (ee); I (aye); O (oh); U (yoo); and "Y (why)" [and sometimes, "Why Not!?"]. *Variants:* 1. For a large group, can come forward as a big cluster of people (not holding hands), raising the (free) arms to the sky. 2. Use vowel sounds from other languages.

Themed Laughter Exercises (the Leader/Anchor
Person tells a story, participants act them out):

Airport & Flight Laughter
   AIRPORT: 1. You're late, run around with bags. 2. Get Boarding Card. 3. Wave goodbye to your bags, disappearing on the conveyor belt. 4. Get onto airplane.
   FLIGHT: Demonstrate: 1. Show emergency exits (in front; behind; to sides). 2. How to operate the seatbelt. 3. Pull down oxygen mask; put on self, then another. 4. How to inflate life jacket (blowing into it)... + 5. Ask (and offer) directions at destination (all in gibberish). 6. Show pictures you took, but you left the lens cap on and they're all blank...

; throw them away, you're free! (etc.)

Household Chores Laughter   Wash dishes; Pass the vacuum cleaner; Clean windows; Fold and iron laundry; etc.

Laughter Revival   A group of laughers finds an unconscious person; in gibberish they argue for a few moments about calling emergency help. "All we need to do is share laughter energy." All place their hands over the person, waving and laughing; the "unconscious" person slowly regains consciousness. All celebrate and continue on together.

Party Laughter   Use several previous exercises: Meet the partygoers (Greeting/Handshake and Namaste); "Oops, I left something at home" (so do Cellphone Laughter); Ate Spicy Food (Hot Soup Laughter).   + Make groups of two's and three's and laugh with each other over imaginary drinks. Have "very amusing", joke-filled conversations - entirely in gibberish.

Floor Laughter Exercises

Belly Laughter   Lie down on your back, bodies at right angles (with your head on another's belly, and someone else's head on your belly).   Let the laughter out!

Bull's Eye Laughter (aka "Sunflower Laughter")   On the back, lie on the floor, heads towards the center of the circle, feet out towards the periphery (looking like the petals of a flower, or a target). Do **Laughter Meditation** (eyes closed, laughing for no reason).

Centipede Laughter (aka "Zipper") Lie in a line on the floor, everyone on their back. The first person has their head to the center and their feet to the right; the next person puts their head adjacent to the first person (their head towards the center) but their feet to the left. (Your head is right next to that of the next person, while their body extends away in the direction opposite your own body). *Variants:* 1. Kick legs like riding a bicycle in the air. 2. Arms up, hold/touch others' hands. 3. Hold knees close to chest. 4. Arms up; kick legs and shake the arms/waggle the fingers of the outstretched hands. 5. Sit back-to-back, elbows interlocked. 6. Sit back-to-back, cross arms in front, take the hand of the person to either side (or behind you); do side-to-side handshakes.

Rowing Laughter Sit straddling others, arms in front; pretend you are rowing a boat, "Aeee; aeee..."; after 2 to 4 times, lean back and howl, resting on the belly of the person behind you.

Bonus Laughter Exercises

Gibberish Punchlines (from Laguna Laughter Club) One person tells, entirely in gibberish, the last few words of a pretend "joke". When they finish, everyone laughs like it was hysterically funny (can "fall down laughing" if desired); congratulates and praises the "joke teller"; nudges each other at how funny it was, how lucky they are to be there to hear such a great joke, etc. Let 4 or 5 people have a turn. *Variation: "One-Word Gibberish Punchlines"* Everyone raises their arms and inhales; one person says a *single* word, in gibberish; everyone laughs like it was hysterically funny (other reactions as above). After 5 to 10 seconds laughing, go around to the next person who gets to deliver the One-Word Punchline.

Gratitude Laughter (aka "Doctor Kataria Laughter") Arms at thigh level with palms facing forward, chest open. Walk around; whatever comes into your awareness, greet it with open-hearted unconditional laughter, acceptance and gratitude. Include people, plants, animals, clouds – whatever, and *everything*, which is in your environment.

Hearty Laughter Feet are shoulder-width apart. Spread your arms up to the sky, tilt your head back and let out a big laugh which shakes your whole heart.

Fundamental Practices

"Ho, ho, ha-ha-ha" Clapping and chanting to "cha cha" rhythm - one, two, one-two-three. Make eye contact, bend knees, place hands to one side and then the other, walk around, do dance-like movements, etc.

"Very Good, Very Good; Yay!" Clap, clap; raise arms up above head in joy. 1. Thumbs up, fingers in a gentle fist; 2. Fingers spread wide. Do in many languages: "Tres bien, tres bien, Ouai!", "Muy bien, muy bien, Orale!", etc.

Relaxation Scan the entire body, consciously relaxing each and every body part.

Breathing Exercises

Breathe in very deeply. On the first repetitions, breathe out quietly, extending effort to exhale as deeply as possible, emptying the lungs. On the later repetitions, laugh aloud in the place of the exhalation.

1. Arms Up The Front Start with hands down by the sides, fingertips towards the earth. On the inhale, raise arms high up above the head (palms face forward).   Lower arms slowly on the exhale.

2. Hastasana (or Tadasana Urdhva Hastasana) (Arms Stay Above Head) First, bring arms up above the head, place palms together. Inhale and exhale while keeping the arms up.

3. Reverse Prayer (or Butterfly Wings or 'Montalbanasana') Bring backs of fingers together in front of the chest (thumbs toward sky); then hands go up and behind the head, fingers pointing down towards the earth (behind the back). Stretch elbows wide apart; inhale and exhale, keeping arms in position.

4. Arm Stretch (aka "Salutation To The Fun") Interlace fingers below the waist, palms facing the belly. While inhaling, raise the arms up: palms to the face, then rotate the palms forward and up, ending with palms directed to the sky. Take a big stretch, continuing to inhale deeply ---"Hold it, hold it..." --- release the hands as you exhale, lowering the arms gradually down to the sides.

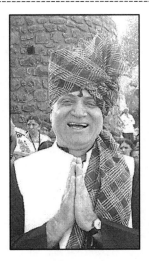

Laughter Exercises

Titles © 2007 Doctor Kataria School of Laughter Yoga

Descriptions (and Breathing Exercise Titles) © 2008, 2011 Jeffrey Briar, The Laughter Yoga Institute

More Laughter Exercises

(added by Dr. Kataria 2015-2016)

Aches and Pains Point to, or place hands on, an area where you've ever felt an ache or pain (foot, knee, back, neck, head, teeth, etc.). "Boo hoo" a moment, then laugh aloud. Continue, indicating several other areas (sympathizing with others).

Airplane (original: p. 32)
Bird Variation: Chicken Laughter (original: p. 27)
Guru (original: pp. 28-29)

High Five Raise one arm with palm facing away; slap another's hand: "Give me five!"

Magic Laughter Extend the arms in front, hands as fists. Raise the pointer fingers of both hands. Tap the inside edge of the hands together, saying "Ay" (pronounced as in "day"). Separate them, then bring together again with "Ay". The third time, raise two fingers (the pointer and middle fingers) up on each hand, as if you've made them magically multiply. "Ha haaa – I did magic!"

Milkshake Variations (original: pp. 30-31)
a) After combining the two cups, you begin to drink; it tastes funny, so
   i. pour the milkshake out (over your head and behind your back); and/or
   ii. pour it out on the earth in front of you.

b) Share the milkshake with others by pouring it down the back of their shirt, tossing above their head, etc.

Sports Theme Pretend to be participating in any desired sport: Juggling, Basketball, Baseball, Football, Sumo Wrestling, Weightlifting, Javelin Throwing, Soccer, Water Polo, etc. Exaggerate the moves - take deep breaths, which turn into laughter.

Waxing Laughter Pretending to place wax on the arms, move one palm over the other arm from elbow to wrist. One application with "Ay"; a second application, "Ay…" The third time, pull from wrist to elbow, as if stripping off the wax, yell "Ah- ha ha ha ha!" It feels great to tear that hair out with laughter!

Wi-Fi Laughter Have the hands by the upper sides of the head. Make fists but with the pointer finger extended. Walk around, seeking a Wi-Fi network connection… when you find one, "Ha ha!"

Zoo Animal Theme Each person walks around acting like any animal they choose (Elephant, Lion, Kangaroo, Monkey, Snake, Chicken, Penguin, Duck…). Can change to another animal whenever desired.

When Dr. Kataria published a revised list of Foundation Exercises in 2015, the following had been removed: American Cowboy, Calcutta, Crying, Royal, Hot Sand, Hugging, Milk Curd, Orchestra, Creative.

Some of the World's Favorite Laughter Exercises

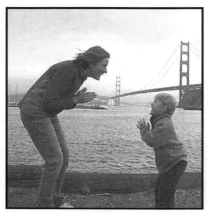

Namaste

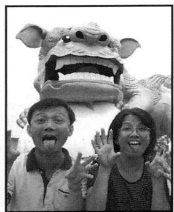

Lion

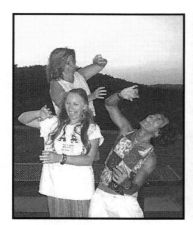

Milkshake

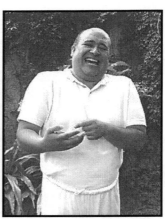

Credit Card Bill

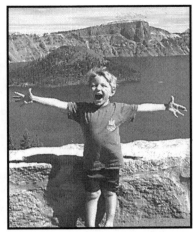

Hearty

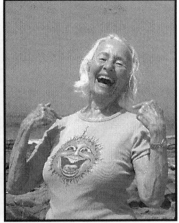

Laugh at Yourself

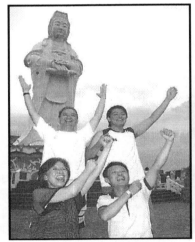

One Meter

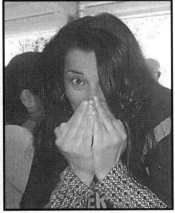

Shy

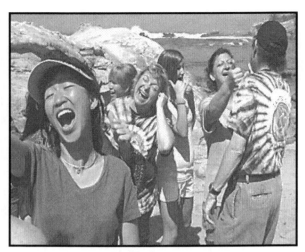

Cellphone

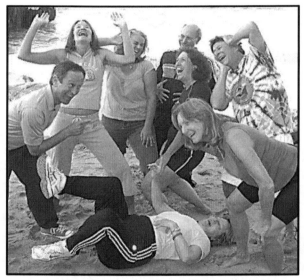

Gibberish Punchlines

From The Laughter Yoga Institute – Compiled by Jeffrey Briar
www.LYInstitute.org ~ Info@LYInstitute.org

Encouraging Words

During laughter sessions, as an exercise concludes, let the air resound with comments like these. Words of encouragement remind the participants that they are in a supportive atmosphere where their playfulness is genuinely welcome. The Critical Mind can be calmed by the assurance that the person's actions are greeted with acceptance, even to the point of gratitude and celebration. This will encourage continued participation (rather than the individual withdrawing to listen to the judgments of their Inner Critic).

As you complete an exercise, call out a word (or several) of encouragement before moving on. Deliver them with enthusiasm!

Just *reading* these will make you feel good.
Hint: put them up on your bathroom mirror or refrigerator. Read often - let yourself accept the praise!

[In the following, the implied exclamation points (!!) are deleted to make the reading less tiring.]

Encouraging Words

Some favorites:

- Great job!
- Alright
- Oh, yeah
- Super job, gang
- Fantastic
- Brilliant
- Wonderful
- You're doing great
- Uh huh, uh huh; That's the way I like it
- Perfect
- Beautiful!

Other great exclamations:

Absolutely - - -!
(Absolutely amazing, absolutely fantastic, etc.)
A-plus job, everybody
Awesome
'Best aerobic workout in the world
Best in the West
Bingo
'Bit of alright
Boing
Bravissimo
Bravo
Classic
Cowabunga
Cragzap
Deee-lectable
Deee-licious
Deee-lightful!
Deee-lovely!
Dynamic
Dynamite
Dynamo
Excellent
Exemplary
Fabulous
Fantabulous
Feelin' good
Feel so good, feel so fine
Fun fun fun
Get down
Get funky
Go--- (Go laffers; go girlfriend; go surfers, etc.)
Google-icious
Great
Hallelujah
Happy days are here again
Healthier and healthier
Healthy, happy,
Howsabout it
Hinky dinky parlay voo
Hip hip hooray
Hoo-ray
Hooray for Captain Spaulding
Hot-cha-cha
Hot dog
Hubba hubba
Hunga dunga
I adore (love) this
I love what you do to me
I love (adore) you!

Immune system --- is
happy! (Lungs are happy;
Feet, Heart, Knees, Toes,
etc.)
I'm proud of us
I'm ready to go
Incredible
I still respect you
It's never too late to
have a happy childhood
I want fries with that
Joy to the world
Knock me out
Let it out
Let it loose
Let it be
Lookin' Good (Fine)
Loosenin' up
Magnificent
'Makes me feel so
good
Marvelous
Masterfully done
Now we're flying
Now we're havin' fun
Now we're takin' off
Now we've got it
Ooh baby that's what I
want (- what I like)
Original
Outstanding
Phenomenal
Priceless
Rama lama ding-dong!

Really---! (Really good,
really awesome, etc.)
Remarkable
Right on
Rock and Roll
Sensational
Shake it, baby
Shake it up
Shazam
Sock it to me
So much to be grateful for
Spectacular
Speechless
Supercalifragialistic...
Super-duper
Terrific
Thank you
Thankyou-thankyou-
thankyou
That makes me happy
That's right
That's the best
That's the way to do it
That was special
There's no stoppin' us
now
This is soooooo good
Totally - - - (Totally
excellent, Totally right-
on, etc.)
--- to the max (Super
to the max, Cowabunga to
the max, etc.)
Way down upon the
Swanee River!

'Way to go!
We are all in this together
We are *doin'* it
We are one
We are together
We be friends
We have got it together
We're free
We're healthy
We're not in Kansas any more
We're on top of the world
We're on our way
We're reelin' and rockin'
Well done
What a gift
What a great workout
What a marvel
What a treasure
What a treat
What good listeners
What you say
Whoo-ie
Whoopie
World-class
Wowie
Ya-hoo
Yee-haw
Yee-ow
Yippie
You hound dogs
You've got friends
You've got it!

Special thanks to **Dr. Catherine Maloof** whose compilation of "Words to Praise Children" greatly inspired the above collection.

Guided Relaxation Scripts

Some of the benefits of a laughter session are achieved only when we include a period of relaxation. The immune system specifically requires a time of rest in order to recharge itself. Even when we are engaged in healthy exercise such as walking, jogging, or playing a pleasurable sport, the immune system is "on hold". It is when we sleep at night, or take a nap, that the immune system rebuilds itself.

However, we often don't get as much sleep as we'd like to, or we don't get that important mid-day nap. So include a period of rest near the end of a laughter session. Thus the participants can receive all the health benefits of laughing.

Following are simple guided relaxation scripts of varying durations. Always speak slowly and include many pauses. During these silent times the listener can relax more deeply.

1. Deep Relaxation
(Five to Ten Minutes)

GETTING INTO POSITION
"Bring yourself to a comfortable position, seated, or standing with your weight evenly balanced. We're going to go over the body from inside, directing every body part to relax more and more deeply.

Ideally, the body will become so relaxed, it's as if the body was falling asleep. At the same time, the mind - the awareness - will still be quite present, quite alert; watching as the body becomes more and more relaxed."

DIRECT THE RELAXATION

"Bring your awareness to your toes. Of both feet, give the toes a gentle wiggle... then let them relax. Mentally, tell your toes to relax, and enjoy the feeling of the toes relaxing, relaxing; the toes are completely and totally relaxed.

Now bring awareness to the feet, and let go of any tension or holding in the feet. Allow the feet to completely relax. Bring the awareness to the ankles, and let the ankles relax. Direct the awareness to the shins and calves; allow them to relax. The knees and kneecaps, relax. The upper leg and thighs, inside and out: all the thighs relax. The thigh socket, in the pelvis: relax.

Now all the feet and legs are completely and totally relaxed.

Bring the awareness to the pelvic area. Let the buttocks muscles, the pelvis, and the hips relax. All the muscles, bones, and organs, of the hips and inside the pelvic area: relax.

Now the low spine; the low back; relax. The belly and intestines, relax. Bring the awareness to the middle spine; the middle back; relax. The abdomen

and solar plexus: relax. Awareness now to the upper
spine and upper back: relax. The upper spine, the
shoulder blades, relax. The back of the rib cage, the
sides of the ribs; the front of the rib cage: relax. And
the chest: relax. Inside the rib cage, the organs inside:
relax. The lungs and heart, relax. The liver and
stomach: relax. The kidneys and adrenal glands: relax.
All the torso and all the inner organs, relax.

Now all the torso, and organs inside, are
completely and totally: relaxed.

Direct the awareness to the armpits and
shoulders. Let the armpits and shoulders: relax. Upper
arms and elbows: relax. Forearms, wrists: relax. The
hands, the fingers, let go; hands and fingers: relax.

All the arms, hands, and fingers are now
completely and totally relaxed.

Direct the awareness now to the tops of the
shoulders, and let the shoulder tops: relax. Enjoy the
feeling of the shoulder tops relaxed.

Now the neck and throat; let go, released; neck
and throat: relax. Awareness now to the mouth; the
tongue relaxed, the teeth: relaxed. The lips; the jaw;
the ears: relaxed. The temples, the back of the head:
relax. The cheeks of the face; the sides of the nose:
relax. The nose, relax; the sinuses: relax. The eyes; let
go the eyes. The eyes are: relaxed. Eyebrows: relax.
Forehead: relax; scalp, and hair: relax; all the head:
relaxed. The skull bones: relax. The brain: relax.

Now all the head, muscles, skull-bones, and even the brain, are completely and totally relaxed.

Even let "thinking" be relaxed. The mind: let go, let the thoughts just evaporate. Knowing that any truly important thoughts will return later, for now, let the mind just release. "Mind" becoming empty, peaceful and calm; "Mind": relaxed.

Take a few moments now just to rest, the body relaxed, the mind relaxed; just being. Being in the present moment, resting in the present moment; being at peace, feeling oneness with all of life."

RETURNING TO EVERYDAY CONSCIOUSNESS

"Beautiful. Now gently bring your awareness - to the breath. Feel the breath flowing in, the breath flowing out.

To bring back awareness of the body, let's choose to take a big breath in. Do that now: big breath in --- then let it out, relax. Now let's start to wake up the body: wiggle the fingers, move the hands; the wrists; the elbows. Move the shoulders, the arms.

Now move the mouth, the lips, the jaw; the tongue, the face. Move the neck and the head around a little bit. Now move the toes of the feet, and now the legs. With the feet on the floor, move the pelvis; the back, the hips... move everything now; wiggle, fidget, stretch --- take another big breath in, inhale deeply and --- let it go, relax.

Now if you're on the floor, gently roll to one side, and pressing your hands against the floor for support, come on up to sitting.

Guided Relaxation has ended."

Allow a few moments for people to reorient themselves to again sitting upright.

Now is a good time for gently sharing announcements, receiving comments; people can share from a centered and peaceful place.

Refreshed and relaxed, please enjoy the rest of your day!

… … … …

2. *Brief* Guided Relaxation
(Three to Five Minutes)

"Bring your awareness to your toes. Give the toes a gentle wiggle; allow the toes to: relax. Tell your toes to relax, and – enjoy the feeling of the toes, relaxed.

Now all the feet: let go of any tension or holding in the feet. Let the feet: relax.

The lower legs, knees, and thighs; all the legs, release. All the legs are: relaxed.

Now the pelvic area, hips; all the organs and muscles inside the pelvic area: relax.

Low back, low spine, belly: relax. Middle back, middle spine, abdomen: relax.

Upper spine, upper back, chest: relax. And all the organs inside the chest: relax... relax... relax. All the torso, and inner organs, are now completely, and totally: relaxed.

Bring the awareness to the armpits and shoulders, and let the armpits and shoulders: relax. All the arms, wrists, hands and fingers: relax. Let them go; arms and hands are completely, and totally: relaxed.

Direct the awareness now to the shoulder tops, and let the tops of the shoulders: relax.

The neck and throat: relax. The jaw, the mouth, the lips: relax.

The ears, temples; the back of the head: relax. The face, the nose, the eyes: relax.

Eyebrows, forehead... scalp and hair: relax.

All the head, and the brain: relax. Now all the head is completely, and totally: relaxed.

With the body relaxed, bring the awareness to the Mind.

Watch the Mind, and allow the Mind to: relax. Knowing that any truly important thoughts will return later, allow the thoughts to dissipate into nothingness, "Like pieces of cloud dissolving in sunlight." Mind released, peaceful; Mind calm... Mind: relaxed.

With Body and Mind relaxed, take a few moments to simply rest in the present moment. Resting in oneness with all of life.

...

(*To come out of the relaxation*) :

Lovely. Beautiful. Gently now, bring the awareness back to the breath. We're going to link our mind and body through the breath. In a few moments, we're going to choose to take a big breath IN, together. Let's do that now. Take a big breath in – – – and let it out, release that breath completely.

Continue to breathe deeply in, and out, as we start to wake up the rest of the body.

Wiggle the fingers, move the hands; move the arms, shoulders; stretch the face; move the neck and head around. Move the feet, the legs; move the back; move everything. Stretch, wiggle, shake – – – take in another big breath… and let it all go, relax.
Gently come back to sitting."

...   .

3. *Quick* Relax
(One Minute)

To be spoken very slowly. The word "relax" might sound more like: "Reeee--laaaaaxxxx…" (the expression of that word lasting 5 seconds). Take a pause after every " : " and " ; " and longer pauses after every " . "

The speaker's voice would give a sense of relaxation, release, and profound peace.

Version A: From Head to Toe

"Bring the awareness to the space above the head. A wave of relaxation is going to descend from above. As we become aware of a body part, that part will immediately relax.

And, here we go:

The top of the head: relax.

The eyes; the ears; the mouth; all of the head: relax.

Let that wave of relaxation descend; the neck and throat: relax.

The shoulders; the arms, hands, and fingers: relax.

The chest, the belly, and all the organs inside: relax.

The hips and pelvis, and all the organs inside: relax.

Let go completely.

The upper legs, the knees: relax. The lower legs, ankles: relax.

The feet, the toes: relax.

All the body now, completely and totally: relaxed."

...   .

Version B: From the Toes to the Top of the Head

"A wave of relaxation is going to rise up our body. As we become aware of a body part, that part will immediately relax.

And, here we go:

The toes; the feet: relax.

The lower legs, the ankles: relax.

The knees, relax. The upper legs: relax

The hips and pelvis, and the organs inside: relax.

Let go completely.

The chest; the belly; and all the organs inside: relax.

The shoulders; the arms, hands, and fingers: relax.

The neck and throat: relax.

The mouth; the ears; the eyes; all of the head: relax.

The top of the head: relax.

All the body now, completely and totally: relaxed."

Creating Your Own (Solo) Laughter Practice

(J. Briar)

To have Laughter change your life, you'll want to practice every day until it becomes a habit. This should take about 40 days. It is *best*, and easiest, to laugh in the company of others, but on days when you cannot get to a club or a group of supportive friends, you can play with this suggested solo practice.

Feel free to improvise and change so that it works for you. If you are laughing heartily and feeling good for 15-20 minutes, you've DONE it!

PREPARATION: All-Over Body Warm-Up.

Easy stretches and swings (try rotating each joint through its full range of motion, trying to gently increase the range, while breathing deeply). 5-10 minutes.

BREATHING AND LAUGHING:

1) Three Pranayama Breathing Exercises, lifting the arms. In each: INHALE for a slow count of 4, HOLD and stretch for a count of 2, and EXHALE for a count of 6, consciously pushing the air out and squeezing the lungs empty at the end. Repeat each practice 4 times before moving onto the next.

a. Arms rise up in front, lowering while exhaling.

b. Arms up and to sides with palms together above the head; arms remain up as you exhale.

c. Butterfly Wings ("Reverse Prayer") behind head; arms remain as you exhale.

2) Now do the same three exercises, but LAUGH while exhaling : four laughing breaths in each position.

3) Kapalabhati ("Bellows Breath") - firm pumping in of the abdomen as breath goes out through the nose, then release abdomen and breath is naturally drawn in: 10-30 times slowly, 20-30 times faster, 10-20 times slowly. (Rest.)

4) Lion Pose (silently).

5) Repeat Kapalabhati, and then Lion Pose.

6) Kapalabhati with "Ho, Ho; Ha, Ha" on exhalation (also known as "Calcutta Laughter"). First gently, then louder, then softer, then silently/only breath. Play with different levels of volume and speed. About 40-60 times.

7) Lion Laughter (on exhale: at beginning of exhalation, growl; then turn into laughter).

8) Repeat Kapalabhati with "Ho, Ho; Ha, Ha" and "Lion Laughter".

9) **Laughter Exercises: your choice – 12 to 20 minutes. Suggestions: "Namaste"/Greeting Laughter (done to furniture, pictures, distant objects), Hearty Laughter, Argument, Forgiveness, One Meter, Cell Phone, Shy, etc. (pp. 26-39). Pick your favorites – also try variety/new exercises.**

The following as suggested by Dr. Kataria in May, 2005:

10) Humming Breath: 12-15 times.

11) Meditate on Silence: 2-3 minutes.

12) "Om" Mantra (15-20 repetitions, different tones).

13) Quiet Meditation (awareness on the breath) – 5-10 minutes.

14) Pray for (or visualize) peace and joy: for your family, friends, teachers, students, people you like and admire, people who have hurt you, strangers; your city, state, country, the earth, and the entire universe.

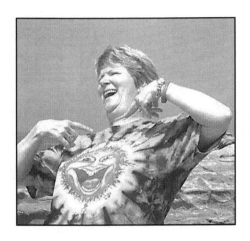

Also see the Laughter Yoga Leader and Teacher Manuals for suggested techniques to develop a "Laughing Alone" practice.

"Take the Laughs On The Road"
(Driving-in-the-Car Laughter)

Laughter *en route* can make driving more pleasurable than you've ever imagined. Of course, **you must be prepared to discontinue laughing any time, and to always maintain enough composure to drive safely and with control.** Nonetheless, you *can* laugh and drive at the same time, and enjoy every minute of it.

It is perhaps most important to develop and allow the blossoming of the *inner* sense of Joyfulness, celebration, laughter and happiness. This is easier to do than making big movements or laughing with complete and "reckless" (?!?) abandon.

The goal, as with any good laughter session, is to laugh for 15 to 20 minutes. To begin, look at your car's clock or your wristwatch and start laughing away. After about 30 seconds take a rest for 15 to 20 seconds. Stretch your arms, back, shoulders, or other body parts (but keep your hands on the steering wheel, and your eyes on the road); take some deep breaths. Then do another round of laughter. You will need about 15 exercises to laugh for 15-20 minutes. Repeat your favorites! You'll be surprised how fast the time will joyously pass.

If there are others in the car, invite them to laugh with you. This will make it much easier for you (and everyone) to laugh, and more pleasurable for all, as well as bonding you in a friendly and pleasant way, and creating gratitude, mutual happiness... and quite possibly an unforgettable memory of a most enjoyable shared drive.

Laughter Practices
You *Can* Do Safely in a Car

Breathe in deeply, hold a few seconds, then **laugh that breath out.** Repeat from time to time, experimenting with different kinds of laughter out: soft giggles, big loud guffaws, medium chuckles, etc.

    Gradient: giggle softly, grow into laughing moderately, expand into huge guffaws – then flow back and forth between various levels

    Gibberish Argument

    Gibberish "I Love You, Ooo Baby!" (as if in a porno movie)

    Gibberish joke-punchline, and reaction

    Slumber Party (suppressed laughter)

    "Naughty Naughty," Cellphone, Jackpot, Royal, Appreciation (one hand at a time)

    Lion Laughter (just the facial expression, without hands); **many other Laughter Exercises** (always keep your hands on the steering wheel)

    Laugh at other cars ("because of" their color, design, license plate meaning – or no meaning; their wheels turning, how they reflect the light, or any other "reason" that occurs to you – or for no reason at all) [NOTE: Refrain from laughing at other drivers, as they may, if they see you, wonder why you are laughing "at them," and as they try to figure out why, they may drive unsafely.]

Laugh at Billboards (no matter what they say), every time you see one

Laugh at Anything/everything as it appears: restaurants, road signs, motels, rocks, off-ramps, telephone poles; the color yellow, red, white, black – as soon as you become aware of it, laugh

Mad Scientist/Maniac ("BRU-ha-ha-ha-ha!")

Body Parts ("Find The Laugh") – point to, touch, or just imagine pointing to a place on your body (knee, belly button, nose, elbow, etc.) and laugh at each one. "I love my knee : ha ha ha ha ha! I love my shoulder : Hee hee hee," etc. No need to look (keep your eyes on the highway!), just know, or think of, the place to which you are indicating.

Laugh Songs: "Ode to Joy", "Funiculi Funicula", "Jingle Bells", "Hallelujah Chorus", "Old McDonald Had a Farm", etc. – laughing instead of saying words

Sing the Laughin' Blues, especially good if there are two or more people. One sings the first phrase, in gibberish or laughter, the other sings the repeat of that phrase. Think of "St. Louis Blues" or something by The Blues Brothers. Also: trade off being saxophones, trumpets, trombones, drums, backup singers – all in laughter and gibberish.

Laughter Exercises for the Blind

(Refer to pp. 26-42)

One Meter

Milkshake

Santa Claus

Mad Scientist

Royal – follow with:

      Oktoberfest (Rowdy Drinking Buddies)

Vowel sounds

Gradient (low to high to low; no hands)

Play with a Ball – toss up, bounce, balance on one finger, spin on head

Jackpot

Gibberish Punchlines (touch –or name- one person to cue them to deliver the Gibberish)

Follow the Leader (sound-wise)

Wicked Witch - follow with:

      Good Witch - follow with:

            Good Witch/Bad Witch

Working with Seniors

Reflections after nine years doing Laughter Yoga with Elders

"People today are living longer and staying healthier than any generation before. The gift of extra years in adulthood means people have more time for personal growth. " -- Emilio Pardo, executive Vice President of AARP (Association of American Retired Persons)

1. Elders are people, too.

Folks in their senior years are just regular folks. They're not necessarily disabled or extra-frail. Many Elders are still quite fit, playing tennis, surfing, swimming, mountain biking, running marathons, jogging 5 (or 10, or 50) miles.

That said, let me hasten to add: Most people, once they've passed the age of 30, have sustained

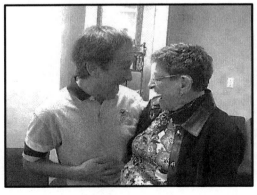

some injuries, whether from a sports accident or stepping off a curb. This may result in some minor disability: a recurring sore back, shoulder pain, stiff knee, etc. Elders by definition have had more time to collect life experiences, including physical mishaps. You may find that, as a group, they have a relatively high percentage of minor (or major) physical challenges. When you first meet a new group of Elders, consider it an opportunity to learn what their life experiences have been, and what limitations they have, *if any*.

Some have challenges, but their situations may be very unique. One may have a non-functional shoulder, while their mind is sharp as that of a teenager. Another may be physically fine but has substantial memory loss. Another may be mentally alert but lost lung function, so they can't breathe as deeply as they'd like.

Elders are not inherently handicapped people. They don't need to be coddled or talked down to. They just need to be treated with *consideration*, and respect, as all people do.

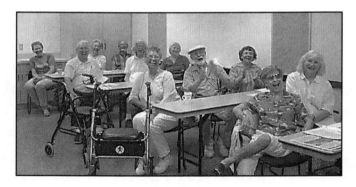

Anticipating there may be some with physical challenges, be prepared with plenty of chairs for them to sit in. Advise the participants that it's okay to sit, stand, change positions, etc. whenever they want to.

They can honor their limitations in advance or at the
moment they become aware of them. Remind
participants that they can modify a practice to fit their
comfort level, sit down if they feel tired, or take a rest.

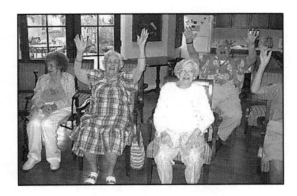

When you work with groups where there is
considerable loss of cognitive functioning (these days,
often folks in their 90s and 100s), then you might
choose to: use music, and sing songs together from
their childhood.

Mix up those who are seated, in chairs or
wheelchairs, with those who can walk around. For
example: place the chair-bound in the center, facing
out; when the Laughter Exercise is in progress, the
Walking Folks can move around and interact with the
chair-bound, as well as their fellow Walking Folks.
Within the time of a few exercises, everyone will be
able to interact with nearly everyone else.

2. Let go of your expectations. Work with where they're at.

Their level of expression may seem low to us more youthful folks. But what we think is "barely moving" may, for them, be the best workout they've had in years.

It is also possible that *some* may romp around the room, frolicking like young deer, or work their way down to the floor and spin around like a child, or a break-dancing teen!

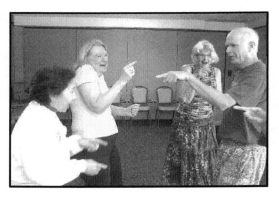

Embrace miracle stories! Don't be surprised if you hear of pain disappearing after decades of suffering, or other amazing tales.

One Laughter Leader recounts doing a session at a senior home where a 74-year-old woman seemed at first skeptical but then joined in heartily – a seemingly unexceptional case. After the session the elder woman came up to the Laughter Leader and thanked her profusely, saying "That's the first time I've laughed in fifty-seven years."

When this woman was 17 years old, she was "slammed". Someone gave her a strong message that laughing out loud was unacceptable.

In Victorian times a socially repressing slogan was: "Ladies smile; only Whores laugh." Any woman who laughed aloud was considered guilty of a crime against good manners, subject to severe stigma and negative judgment. Thus women learned to suppress the expression of joy which had seemed so natural when they were young.

What a blessing to be the Laughter Leader who was able to set this woman free from that negative garbage! Finally, at age 74, she could begin enjoying one of life's great treasures: hearty hilarity shared with caring friends.

3. Look deeply into their eyes. Connect with them. Share from your heart.

When you look into another's eyes, even through cataracts or dimness you can see there's a spark in there, a Child Within; an Inner Five-Year-Old ready to come out and play in a timeless way, even if the body can't keep up with the spirit. They will be so happy to play in spirit (emotionally), they aren't going to focus on the way their body can't participate as fully as it used to.

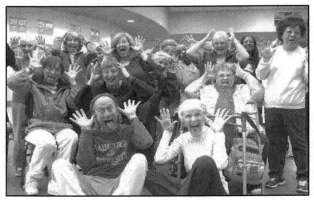

My sincere advice: Get Over Yourself - your self-assessing Critical Mind. If an inner voice gives you a limiting thought such as: "I can't relate to these folks, they're too old/ill/messy", first *thank* your Mind for trying to protect you, and then *move forward* into a Higher Good: sharing and caring for lovely, loving people who just happen to have more years, and injuries, than you have...at least, so far!

Let your heart open. Befriend them unconditionally. Let loving Elders - despite cataracts, or limping legs, or drooping eyelids, or low energy levels - support you in being willing to love anyone and everyone. They'll be glad you did; and *you'll* be glad you did!

... A Love Story:

Ron Dick was in his eighties when we met and began our friendship. His body couldn't do a whole lot. He'd survived many surgeries, and "died" (and was revived) on several occasions. But his mind was acute, his wit brilliant. We roared in laughter at many a joke, devised by either one of us.

Our buddy-hood began before I encountered Laughter Yoga. I was teaching a Chair Exercise class at the senior home where he lived (and where he met his future wife). Ron and I soon came to admire our shared sense of humor. When I brought Laughter Yoga to our friendship, Ron was bemused and intrigued, and happy for me - even though it wasn't his cup of tea. He was glad I didn't give up my sense of humor and ability to create puns, even when I didn't need them anymore in order to laugh.

Ron passed away about 6 years after we'd first met, but we enjoyed a wonderful and mutually enriching friendship while he was here.

And hey, I had a *marriage* which didn't last that many years!

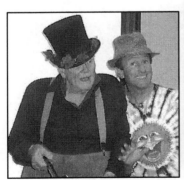 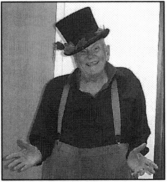

Rascally Ron Dick (we're both "into" hats)

4. Focus on Success, always.

[Thanks to Ruthe Gluckson for her unflinching focus on this aspect of working with all ages – from young children through people with all kinds of disabilities and handicaps to adults in the later years of life.]

Genuinely give attention to and acknowledge their achievements. Examples: "You got one arm off your lap today Marian – great job!" "Hey Bob, I think I actually heard your laugh all the way from the other side of the room here. Well done, pal!" This is not to be sarcastic or fake; it is to sincerely find the victories in each moment's expression.

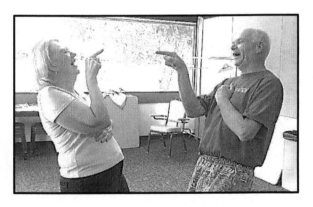

A person's effort can only be judged a "failure" if you've set up a standard which is not met. If you lower expectations - or have *no* expectations, but rather treat every session as a clean slate - then *every* expression, every presence, every positive effort – *even a thought* - is a victory.

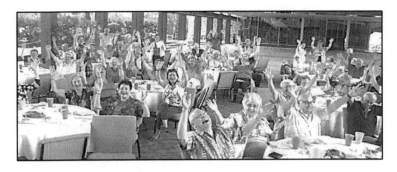

Why Laughter Yoga is so great for Elders.

Laughter brings Joy to life – and everyone *can* do it. Not every Elder can stand up to do Tai Chi, or have the patience to do Meditation. Sometimes, prescribed medications make it nearly impossible to sit still and meditate. Many Elders will not have the coordination to play Ping Pong, or the mental acuity to remember the rules to a card game.

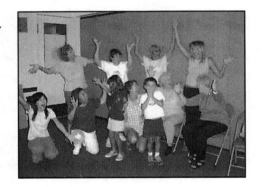

But *everyone* can laugh; nearly everyone can look into another person's eyes, and allow another person to look into their own, and reconnect with the Joy which they felt when they were a child. Such Joy is the birthright of every human being. We can conjure up that same Joy through playful interactive laughter.

So if you are drawn to the idea of working with Elders, or even if you consider it a challenge, my advice is: *Go For It!* Give it a try. You have little to lose, other than your own preconceptions, and much to gain: the Joy - and great stories from the experiences - of a tremendous group of caring, sharing people.

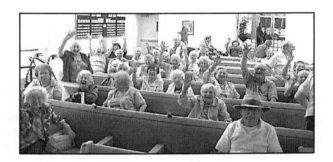

Jeffrey Briar began leading a weekly Laughter Yoga classes at a senior center in Irvine California USA in 2006. (This class continues to this day.) Another senior center engaged him (weekly) for 2 years. He gives frequent Laughter Yoga programs in Board and Care facilities, Senior Apartments and the like; for various Hospital/Health Support Groups; and gives a monthly presentation (changing venues) on "Laughter for Health" representing the Medicare Benefits Management branch of a mutual-benefit medical group.

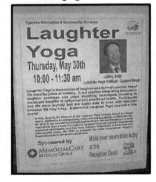

Leading Laughter with Children

Doing Voluntary Laughter with kids is *great*! You can have the most fun, creative, and heart-warming experiences imaginable. You don't need to put on a clown nose, wear funny shoes, or show comedy movies – far from it. Doing "performances" or using props can actually distance you from some kids, putting them into their Critical Mind, as they think "I don't like clowns" or "I already saw that trick" etc. As with all Laughter Yoga, all you have to do is **Be Yourself**, their friendly Laughter Coach, encouraging and supporting them to have fun and enjoy themselves.

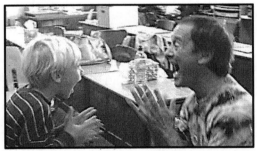

Kids are often the *easiest* to get laughing. Once they realize it is truly okay to have fun and they are not going to be judged as silly or wasting time, they are usually *Ready, Willing and Able* to **Go For It**!

All we need to do is set it up[so they know it's safe to be expressive, and then let them run with the ball.

You do want to give the same advice you'd give to all groups: Take care of yourself (no new pain); play at your own level of comfort, there's no need to "force" anything; we laugh *with* (not "at) each other; and refrain from talking until we're done.

As they get older (12 years or so) it may be helpful to separate them by *Age*, or by *Grade Level*. For example, a High School Senior concerned about how they look in front of their peers may have issues laughing wholeheartedly with a Freshman from the same school. In some cultures, division between genders may also be advisable.

Divide High and Junior High School-age kids into the same grade level or age (so one session would be for "All Sophomores", another would be "All Seniors", etc.). This separating is a judgment call on your part - you may be lucky to find that some kids are perfectly comfortable laughing with other kids of all grades, ages, colors, sizes, etc. This is most often true with those children with experience as babysitters, caregiving or otherwise working with all-ages. It may be wise to err on the side of caution here, especially at first, and keep the adolescent and near-adolescent kids divided into age-specific or grade-specific groups. In this way we alleviate the concerns of their Critical Minds so there is a minimum of evaluating/judging going on, leading to a greater level of participation and fun.

>>> The Top-Recommended Laughter Exercise to have Success in Laughing with Children is:

*** FOLLOW- THE- LEADER. (You go first.) ***

Instructions:

Stand at the front with all the others in a mass, facing you; they are like a standing audience. Everyone would ideally be at the same height level. Instruct the

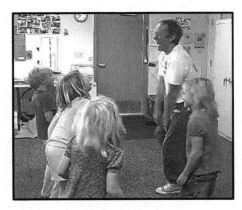

students to copy your movement and laughter style, and that other students will have a chance to lead the rest of us. The children are to imitate the person who is laughing at the front of the room.

Model doing some fun (but not *too* silly) laughter exercises/moves for just a few seconds, such as: Waving, Santa Claus, Penguin, Silent, Milkshake, Hearty Laughter, different kinds of Laughter-Dances, etc. Avoid sexual stereotypes like Striptease Dancer, Macho Weightlifter, etc. After you've been the Leader for about 10 seconds, pick a playful-looking student to come up and take a turn as the next Leader. After this person has done some movements and laughter (while being copied by the others) for 5 to 15 seconds, let them go, by saying something like "Okay; great, Friend! And the next Leader will be…" Then pick another person to come up.

Once they've got the flow of it, you can allow the child who is the Leader of the current exercise to select the next person to come up and be the Leader.

Be sure to manage such choosing so that everyone who wants to will get a turn. If the current Leader is selecting exclusively from their private circle of friends, you can step in at the end of one exercise and say "That's great! Let's be sure that everyone gets a turn - how about you over there?" ...and you select a child from a different part of the room.

Because the kids are choosing their own level of expression, they can be as demure or robust as they wish and are not likely to feel embarrassed. And because the others are just copying the Leader - again at *their own* selected level of enthusiasm or shyness - they are also "in the Power Seat" of their own experience so they need not feel embarrassed or "put on the spot".

Of course, if some child simply does not want to participate, we would honor that, and just move on to the next person.

Other Suggestions:

Teach them "Ho, ho, ha-ha-ha" and use this frequently. Many of them love this, the way everyone returns to something with which they feel comfortable – while continuing to breathe, laugh and interact with the others.

For recurring sessions, you may want to come up with a Theme and choose exercises which support that. Examples; Going on a Picnic, to the Beach, to the Movies, to the Mall, to the Zoo; Things that Happen at School; Sports; Dances, etc.

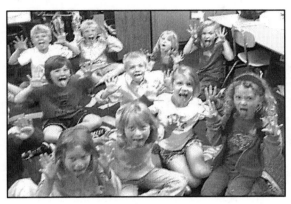

A Guided Relaxation is recommended, if possible, but likely will be short - just a minute or two. You can ask your hosts if they think the kids will be up for a longer relaxation. Be sensitive to your intuition - you might be surprised at how long even 7-year-olds can enjoy closing their eyes and going on an *inner* adventure, becoming aware of their body and feeling everything relax.

Keep your thinking cap on, and a note pad handy! When you support kids in being creative with this much encouragement, some wonderfully brilliant and fun things are likely to occur. You-all may come up with some great new laughter exercises!

Gibberish Made Easy!

Everything you always wanted to know about gibberish - - - not!

In the early days of Laughter Yoga, Gibberish was a warm-up exercise offered to help laughter club members to loosen up their minds and feel more free and playful. Now it has developed into its own form of art and expression.

Some laughter programs dedicate hours, even days, to exploring this technique. The author and Dr. Kataria have produced a *Gibberish Kit* set of 4 full-length videos, available from Laughter Yoga International headquarters in India. The author offers a 2-day training as "Certified Gibberish Coach." See the popular video *Gibberish 101: How to Speak Gibberish* on YouTube.

Gibberish is speaking in nonsense: attempting to express yourself using a "language" which does not make any sense – not to you, nor to anyone else.

Gibberish is about *freedom*! You can "say" anything you want, express any emotion or idea, without fear of being judged or criticized. Since you cannot *be* understood in the first place, there is no danger of being "misunderstood". Thus, you are free to say or express *anything* you'd like.

The suggestions which follow are techniques to get started comfortably to feel loose enough to speak in nonsense-talk. Once you have unlocked the doors to your free expression, forget all these rules, and just let yourself go. Allow the practice of speaking in gibberish to give you the freedom to *let it all out!*

TWO KEYS TO ORIENTATION

Emotions: Entry Point to Free Communication
Imagine you feel strongly about something (or no particular thing). Exaggerate the feeling, and express it with vigor.

Movement: The Key to Communication
Use big, expressive gestures - like you really *mean* what you are saying, emphatically!

TECHNIQUES FOR TALKING NONSENSE

1: One or two word(s) with no meaning "Blah blah blah"; "Yadda yadda, yadda yadd…"; "Bloop blee bloop, blee-blee-blee bloop".

2: Infant-like Speech "Goo goo ga ga gee"; "Bibi booble, doop plurby wurby faw-faw!".

3: A Foreign Language (one you don't actually speak) "Das shinkum varn dee shnowf haffen"; "Zee cwassan say sea boe sez ahnoo".

4: Meaningless Sounds, Body Noises "Cluck, chirp, pbblfft" (flutter tongue, raspberry lips); snorts, coughs, gagging, bird sounds, animal noises.

5: Singing A familiar tune with nonsense words; or sing in gobbledy-gook with no concern for a melody.

6: Backwards Talk As though a film's soundtrack was playing in reverse.

7: Slow Motion Speaking very slowly (not saying real words). "Breeeee– gaaaaw- loooo-oooo- nurrrr…".

8: All Shook Up Mix up any and all styles from above; or whatever comes out (no "real" words, though).

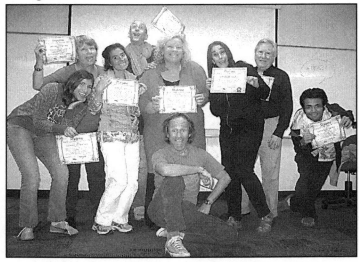

Graduates of a Certified Gibberish Coach training

"Gibberish is a very good tool for developing your creative brain, because in gibberish you don't plan anything, you express spontaneously, on the spot. When you talk in gibberish, you challenge your ideas, your right brain to be more active. Gibberish is an act of playfulness.

"Gibberish can be a very good tool for emotional expression for people, without the need for them to verbalize their feelings." -- Dr. Madan Kataria

The Inner Spirit of Laughter
and the Responsibility Game

When we laugh regularly, free of the need to be reacting to a joke or other reason, we reliably create for ourselves the physiological experience of happiness. But creating happiness for oneself is simply not enough. We need to evoke and nurture what Dr. Kataria calls *The Inner Spirit of Laughter.*

Dr. Kataria recounts how, early in the laughter club movement, a woman called to complain. Her husband was laughing regularly and feeling personally happy, but when he came home he yelled at his wife and family just as he used to do before the laughter club experience. Dr. Kataria realized that the purpose of the laughter club had to be more than merely individual health. The benefits of unconditional laughter needed to spread out into the community. People needed to nurture the *Inner Spirit* of Laughter: desiring and consciously striving to help others to be happy.

This involves not only refraining from getting angry at others, but consciously cultivating attitudes which reflect the peace and joy resultant from a laughter practice.

Kataria encourages laughter club members to pay compliments, and consciously practice forgiveness (*LFNR, pps. 133-149). Steve Wilson codifies the laughter spirit into a 7-days-per-week system he calls

"Good Hearted Living" (*GHL, p.4-6) wherein each day of the week the participant focuses on a positive emotional action: on Mondays paying Compliments, Tuesdays being open-minded and Flexible; Wednesdays cultivating Gratitude. Thursdays are dedicated to performing acts of Kindness; Fridays practicing Forgiveness; and Saturdays and Sundays bringing pleasure and sweetness to one's life (for which Wilson uses the metaphor, "Chocolate").

Laughing Along With Life

The Inner Spirit of Laughter also encompasses the choice of bringing the activity of laughter to whatever happens in our life, as soon as possible. Laughter Club members are encouraged to look at the lighter, easier-to-swallow side of whatever life's circumstances may bring.

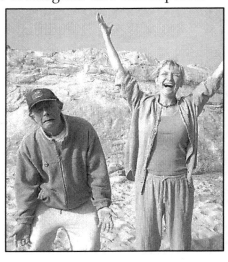

• Drop a plate and see it shatter into a thousand pieces?

Laugh! This is better for your physical and emotional health than berating yourself for your clumsiness, or blaming someone else for placing the plate in an awkward spot, etc.

• Waiting in line at the market, and just before you get to check out, the checker leaves for their lunch break?

Laugh! This is better for your own peace of mind than cursing the hungry checker, or getting angry at the folks in front of you who got served first, etc.

Someone cuts you off in traffic? You discover a stain on your shirt? You lose money in the stock market? If you respond with hostility, you are harming your own physiology. You can instead choose to respond with laughter and acceptance, and when you do, you are improving your health.

Embracing the Inner Spirit of Laughter, we commit to being in a more positive state of mind, ready to laugh at life's inconsistencies and challenges. At the same time, we also bring a more openhearted, accepting attitude to those around us. As we model acceptance of life's challenges, laughing along with them and graciously moving on, perhaps even being compassionate toward others who may be suffering, the attitude of those around us will likewise be elevated. They don't have to handle our complaining or suffering; they can witness a person who responds to disappointment with humor and grace. It can be powerfully impactful on those who witness us as we embrace the Inner Spirit of Laughter.

Voltaire wrote **"God is a comedian, performing for an audience too afraid to laugh"**. When we laugh along with the forces that seem outside of us, we make life seem that much easier to handle.

When Life Gives You Lemons — Make "Laughenade"

The discipline of meeting life's disappointments and challenges with compassionate laughter is practiced (in some of Dr. Kataria's more advanced workshops/trainings) through an exercise called "Ha Ha Mantra", "Life's Little Stresses", or "Free-Floating Hostilities". Your Author sometimes calls this practice "Compassionate Laughter".

Each individual is invited to share with the group something in their life that was an annoyance or cause of stress. Examples: "Just before I wanted to leave to come here, I realized I'd left my car keys at the office." "My boyfriend left the toilet seat up this morning, as usual." "I always seem to spend my whole paycheck before I can take a vacation", etc. After they share this, the rest of the group opens their arms, palms up, and each person lets out a caring and slow "Ha, ha, ha, ha, ha…" (as though to say, "I can relate, I've had similar challenges, too…" or "Oh yes, it can be very frustrating to have such a disappointment. Isn't life unpredictable? Oh well… Ha, ha, ha, ha, ha…"). Each person takes a turn sharing their "stressor" and receiving the compassionate laughter of the rest of the group, The person reporting the stressor is encouraged to laugh along.

As always with this work, there is a sense of laughing "with" - with the vagaries and surprises of life - not "at". We are not laughing "at" the person with the challenge. We are not even laughing "at" the source-of-stress!. We are cultivating the ability to laugh "with" Life, no matter what Life sends us to challenge our composure.

Embracing Responsibility for All of It

Another exercise to cultivate our ability to laugh at things which we might consider stressors is "The 'I'm Responsible For That' Game."

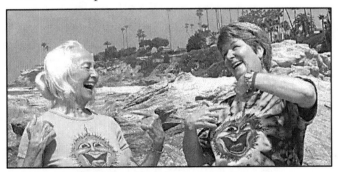

Each participant chooses something that occurred in world history - preferably something important and generally perceived as stressful or "bad" - for which they could not possibly actually be immediately responsible. (Examples: "The Spanish Inquisition", "Slavery in The American Colonies", "The Invention of Money", "The Use of Banned

Pesticides in Third World Countries," "Fleas", etc.)
They say the name of their item, and follow it by
enthusiastically (playfully) saying the phrase, "I'm
responsible for that!" (Example: "The Destruction of
Ancient Rome? I'm responsible for that!")

This is a fun and laugh-provoking practice in
its absurdity, but even more powerful is the next step:
continue to take responsibility for whatever happens,
no matter how absurd it might be to take personal
responsibility for it. In point of fact, we specifically
want to "claim responsibility" for things where it is
unreasonable to do so. Especially: "take
responsibility" for things done by or to others where it
is evident that the responsibility could not realistically
be "yours."

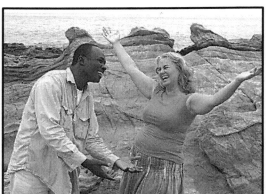

Examples:
Joe: "On my way over here, it started to rain."
Sally (almost interrupting): "Rain? Oh, I'm responsible
for that!"

Kathy: "I heard there was a big traffic jam in the mountains." Sam: "Traffic? I'm responsible for that!", and Brenda steps in with: "And the mountains – I'm responsible for those!"

Shahid: "I love reading about the American Civil War." "David: "War? Oh, (with mock pride) that's my baby!" Corinne: "And reading? That's one of my favorite creations!", etc.

Responsibility as a Choice
Freedom from Guilt

The exercise/game just described can actually make a big impact on us. When things go "wrong" in life, it seems like people (especially in western cultures) are quick to look for "who's to blame?"

• If the train is late, we look for who's responsible, "why" did this happen: was it the fault of the conductor, the scheduler, someone at the previous station whose jacket got caught in the door, etc.

• If the traffic is heavy, we look for who's to blame: the drivers who won't all go the same (faster) speed, the city planners for not building enough freeway lanes, the sporting event a little ahead attracting thousands of additional drivers, or etc.

• Even when it is a Force of Nature, we look for something to blame: There was a tsunami (tidal wave) and a lot of people were killed? "What idiot let them live so close to the ocean; they must not have been praying sufficiently (or perhaps they were living too sinfully); why did they ignore the early warnings (of science, shamans, history, wild birds)", etc.?

We almost never look to the possibility that we ourselves might be "the one to blame" for the current situation.

But what if we did? What if, no matter what Life brought to our awareness – even something from the distant past – what if we greeted everything that came into our awareness with the attitude of: "I am responsible for that!" Not as a source of guilt or shame, but as an exercise in awareness; shifting our typical conditioned response from a negative one (blaming, judging as bad, shifting the blame to another "bad" person or force) to a more positive one (whatever happens, I am responsible – if I created it, this implies that I can handle it).

What occurs is this: very soon, the entire game becomes ridiculous and the negative charge is dissipated. Guilt and shame can be seen as mere mental constructs, and they need not have the iron grip on our attitudes which they otherwise all-too-often do.

Responsibility as a Conscious Practice Bringing Joy to The Party

When we seize responsibility for everything – when we embrace with gusto the game of taking responsibility for all of Life – the absurdity of it all can even get into a comical competition.

Kevin: "I just heard on the news how they want to raise income taxes." Jennifer: "Income taxes? I'm responsible for that!" Doris: "No no, I am!" Jennifer (pouting like a young child): "You got to be responsible for overdue library books! I want "income taxes"!" Doris (also childlike): "Oh, alright this time... you can have income taxes." Jennifer: "Yay! (dancing:) I'm responsible for income taxes, I'm responsible for income taxes!..." Doris: "But next time, I want to be responsible for stubbed toes!...",etc.

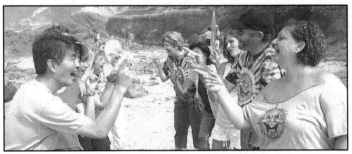

By meeting whatever Life gives us with laughter, playfulness, and childlike innocence - with Joy - our life experience will be more enjoyable, fun and laughter-filled. This will be best for our personal well-being, positive mental attitudes, and spreading the good feelings – the Inner Spirit of Laughter – to all in our world.

* References cited:

   Laugh For No Reason; Kataria, Dr. Madan; Madhuri International publishers, Mumbai/Bombay (India), 1999

   Good-Hearted Living; Wilson, Steve; Steve Wilson and Company publishers, Ohio (USA), 2003

Styles of Learning

Students seeking education come to us with varied backgrounds, from a multitude of training programs and institutions. They may have different ways whereby they best process information; each may have their unique preferred "learning style".

An individual's learning style refers to the ways which work best for them to *Absorb*, *Comprehend*, *Process*, and *Retain* information.

Individual learning styles depend on cognitive, emotional and environmental factors, as well as one's prior experience. In other words: everyone's different.

For example, to learn a laughter exercise some students may get a good understanding by reading printed instructions, while others may learn better by listening to directions on how to do the activity.

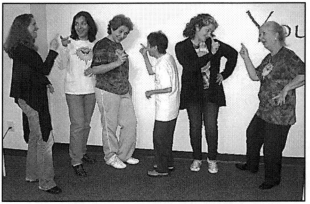

Others will best achieve mastery by the practice of physically performing the exercise with a group.

If students can access information in terms with which they are comfortable, this will increase their academic confidence.

The wise teacher will thus consider *varying* student learning styles when **designing** and **delivering** course content. If we offer a menu (mix) of teaching modalities, content is more likely to be presented in a manner suited to every type of learner. Our students will learn better if we "mix it up" - present information in multiple ways.

Ways People Learn

Education Theory suggests several kinds of learning styles. One of the most popular models, from Fleming and Mills, is referred to as VARK (for "Visual, Audio, Reading/writing, and Kinesthetic/experiential" learners). We've changed the order here to reflect the idea that Laughter Yoga is an experience-based practice.

K Kinesthetic (Do, Experience, Demonstrate; Physical, Tactile)

This modality refers to "the use of experience and practice (simulated or real)." While the method may invoke other modalities, the key is that students learn "through concrete personal experience, examples, practice or simulation." Effective methods include demonstrations, videos and movies, as well as case studies, play-acting and applications.

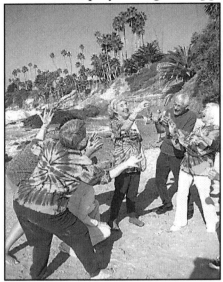

Kinesthetic (tactile) students learn by touch and doing; these are hands-on learners. They present an opportunity to use the senses of movement and touch; you might incorporate physical objects. These learners value their own background of experiences. They also benefit from the experiences of others (although less than when the experience is direct and personal).

Involve Kinesthetic learners in role-playing and active experimentation.

"I see, and I forget. I hear, and I remember.
I do, and I understand." -- Confucius

V Visual (Graphic Representations, See, Watch, Imagine, Picture)

Visual learners prefer the use of images, maps and diagrams. They like charts, graphs, labeled diagrams, illustrations – and symbols like arrows, circles, patterns and shapes.

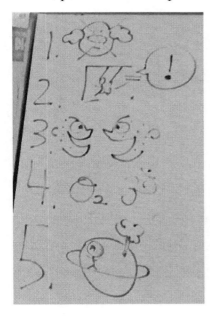

<- A graphic presentation of the 5 Points of "What is Laughter Yoga".

It can be helpful to use a whiteboard and to draw diagrams with meaningful symbols to indicate the relationship between different things. Colors can be used to highlight major and minor links.

Visual learners respond well to how items are laid out – their spatial organization.

A Auditory (Hear, Listen, Speak)

These students prefer information that is heard or spoken. They learn best from lectures, tutorials, sound recordings, group discussions, verbal presentations, and talking things through. Effective speaking may include talking aloud as well as talking to oneself.

Auditory-preferring students may want to sort things out *by* speaking, rather that sorting things out and *then* speaking. They may work best if they have a small group discussion first, prior to speaking to the larger group.

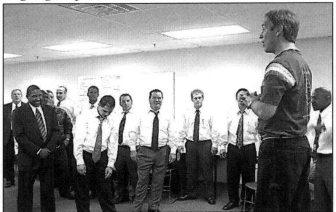

Useful tools include: stories, jokes, music, rhythm, and rhyme.

R Read (Write, Words in Print)

These learners are often avid readers. They prefer to write down information which has been spoken (take notes). Writing will help them remember and conceptualize. These students may turn diagrams and charts *into* words.

Readers sometimes avoid eye contact in order to concentrate. Don't take this personally. They are withdrawing so they can better internalize the information.

Readers may read their notes silently, or read aloud to themselves.

Readers relate well to: manuals, reports, essays, written assignments, and writing summations. Lists and glossaries can be helpful.

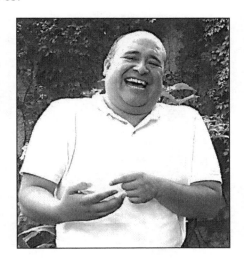

Application

These categories are somewhat arbitrary, and often overlap. Other educational theories direct us to consider additional qualities which may be significant for optimal learning, such as: working solo vs. in a dyad (with a partner) and/or in groups; variations which are cognitive or theoretical; and the manipulation of basic elements in novel ways (being "creative").

Everyone has a mix of learning styles. Some people find that they have a dominant style of learning, with far less use of the other styles. Others may find that they use different styles in different circumstances.

There is no one right mix. Some learners are not satisfied until they have had input in all their preferred modes. They take longer to gather information from each mode, but they then often have a more profound understanding of the topic.

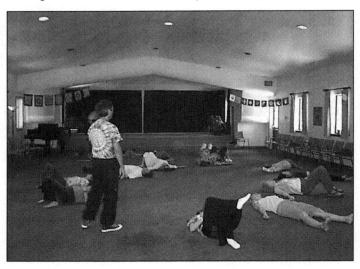

Wrapping Up

Our styles are not fixed. We can develop our capabilities in less dominant styles, as well as further develop styles that we already use well.

Best practice suggests that teachers offer instruction that employs a variety of teaching styles. We would be wise to take into consideration varying styles of learning when we design activities, curriculum and assessments.

Laughter Yoga Exam
(just for fun!)

Written by and © Jeffrey Briar 2011

(ANSWERS will be found on the bottom of p. 153.)

1. Laughter Yoga was

a. Found under a rock in the Brazilian rainforest in 1867

b. Founded by Dr. Madan Kataria, a medical doctor in India, in 1995

c. Described in the *Tibetan Book of the Dead* (pp. 113-119)

d. Invented in a laboratory in Budapest, Hungary in 1942

2. Much of the research on the health benefits of laughter occurred thanks to this popular book by journalist Norman Cousins

a. *A Mighty Wind*

b. *Spartacus*

c. *The Laughing Baby Book*

d. *Anatomy of an Illness - as Perceived by the Patient*

3. Laughter Clubs can be found in approximately how many countries?

a. About a dozen

b. Fewer than seven

c. More than 80

d. Only on the 'Net

4. Laughter Club members have reported improvement with
   a. Depression
   b. High blood pressure
   c. Sleep patterns
   d. Social support
   e. All of the above

5. What is the most important requirement to be able to laugh?
   a. Jokes by Henny Youngman or Eddie Cantor
   b. Willingness
   c. A working video player and films of Charlie Chaplin
   d. Pizza with funny toppings: Anchovies, Cucumber, Broccoli, etc.

6. A good way to become comfortable speaking in Gibberish is
   a. Say one meaningless word repeatedly, like "Blah, blah, blah-blah-blah" while being physically and emotionally expressive
   b. Try to read aloud a book written in a language which you do not understand
   c. Jump out of an airplane and don't allow yourself to say "Geronimo!"
   d. Learn Latin or Greek first

7. Dr. Kataria, the creator of Laughter Yoga, has a first name

a. Madman

b. Mandyke

c. Herschey

d. Madan

8. Laughter Yoga has been featured on which major media?

a. *The Oprah Winfrey Show*

b. *Dancing with the Stars*

c. CNN-TV Special *Happiness and Your Health* with Dr. Sanjay Gupta

d. *Yoga Journal*

e. *The New York Times*

f. All of the above

9. Dr. Kataria's Foundation Laughter Exercises include

a. Shy Laughter

b. Milkshake (originally "Lassi") Laughter

c. One Meter Laughter

d. Lion Laughter

e. All of the above

f. b. and c. only

10. The most effective way to get a group of people to start laughing at the same time is

    a. Use a word with the letter "K", e.g.: "Pickle, Ketchup, Kronkite" (also known as "The Neil Simon Approach")

    b. Tickle their Ants with a Feather (also known as the "Particularly Nasty Weather" technique)

    c. Flip their oxygen tank from O_2 to NO_2 (Oxygen to Nitrous Oxide)(also known as the "Daffy Dentist Protocol")

    d. Give a clear Command to Start, such as: "Are you ready? …Start!" or "Take a deep breath in; and - laugh!" (also known as the "Clear Command to Start" method)

11. Suggested ways to end a Laughter Exercise are

a. Clap the hands while repeatedly chanting "Ho, ho, ha-ha-ha"

b. Raise the arms, show the palms of the hands, and say words of praise and encouragement, e.g. "Great job, everybody," "Fantastic!" etc.

c. Fire a starter pistol and say: "That's it! No more Mister Nice Guy!"

d. Call out "No, stop - you're doing it all wrong," and burst into tears

e. a. and b.

f. c. and d.

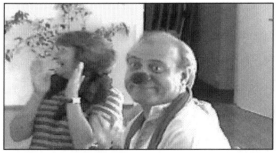

Doctor "Madman"(?) Kataria, 2007

Writing Press Releases
which *ACTUALLY GET PUBLISHED!*
(J. Briar, with special thanks to **Robert Gluckson**)

In the *FIRST PARAGRAPH* of any Press Release, you need to give *most* of the essential information:
* WHAT (Laughter Club meeting)
* WHERE (location in 'your town')
* WHO (presented by Certified Laughter Yoga Leader 'your name here')
* HOW (as in "How to participate"; or often "How Much" = usually in our case, "free!")

This is followed by several paragraphs of information including more details, especially
  * WHY: (Why should I go? What are the benefits, why would someone want to check it out or send a friend)
   Also, more WHAT (just what IS Laughter Yoga), WHO (who created it, who are the leaders), etc.
  Keep this in mind: each, any, or all of the central paragraphs could be omitted and the essential information would still be given – because the vital facts appear in the first and last paragraphs.

The *LAST PARAGRAPH* has a bit more, specifically - like a more exact address/*WHERE*; *and HOW to contact you* for more information.

We must write our Press Releases in the third person, using words like "he, she, they, it." Example: "Laughter Club leader Sally Jones announces…" "Club members report that they feel…"   Do *not* use words like "I and we" (*not*: "We are happy to announce") as this reads like the *newspaper* is presenting the event. But *you* are doing the presentation; the newspaper is simply reporting that someone, not with the newspaper, is doing something. If you send Press Releases with phrases like "*we* are going to have our first session on Sunday…" it is more likely that rather than rewriting it into proper form, the editor will simply discard your release.

If we provide the press release in appropriate form, such announcements are published about one-third to one-fourth of the time. In other words: every three or four times your author has submitted such a press release, one gets published. That's a good average! But don't be discouraged if you send five, ten or twenty before they get printed. You just need to find the perfect time when the paper has the space available. They would prefer to sell that space for advertisements, but if they haven't sold an ad, they can – and *want* to – fill the space with *your* press announcement. By sending regular announcements, even if the "news" is not a large event, the paper gets in the habit of seeing your news and knowing that you exist. Then when you *do* offer a bigger program they are more likely to publish that piece of "bigger" news.

Make up an email list of Media Contacts and send your Press Release to everyone on the list, every time you make up a press release. Obvious recipients are the local newspapers, but you can try *anything* with a "Community Events Calendar": throwaway magazines, respectable papers, sensational newsletters, TV listings, church groups, local blogs and online publications, and neighborhood news - these are actually the BEST.

oOo

Sample Press Release

Contact: Jeffrey Briar   Phone 949 376-1939
Email: info@LYInstitute.org   Web: www.LYInstitute.org

FOR IMMEDIATE RELEASE

Laguna Club now Laughing with the Dolphins
Seven Days per Week

Founder Jeffrey Briar becomes Director of "The Laughter Yoga Institute"

Celebrating the idea that Laughter is the Best Medicine, Laguna
Laughter Club founder Jeffrey Briar announced that the club now
meets seven days per week. The free meetings feature Intentional
Laughter Exercises, without the need for jokes or humor,
combined with yoga breathing techniques and easy stretches.
Briar claims the technique is suitable for all ages and all fitness
levels. Meetings are led by senior student of Dr. Madan Kataria,
the creator of Laughter Yoga. The Laguna Laughter Club meets
daily: Sunday through Friday at 8:00 a.m., and Saturdays at 10:00
a.m. The joyful sounds peal forth on the sand below the gazebo
in Heisler Park, 375 West Cliff Drive in Laguna Beach.

Laughter practices are performed in the fresh open air by the sea.
"It's a great way to start the day with good feelings and an
increased sense of vigor," Mr. Briar said. The Laughter Teacher
claims that laughter's health benefits include: relief from stress,
anxiety, pain and depression; improved circulation, a stronger
immune system; better sleep patterns; a gentle massage to the
internal organs, improving digestion and elimination; enhanced
creativity and increased self-confidence.

The international Laughter Club Movement was founded in 1995 by
Dr. Madan Kataria, a medical doctor in India, and his wife
Madhuri, a Yoga teacher. Dr. and Mrs. Kataria developed "Hasya
Yoga" (Laughter Yoga), which combines the scientific benefits of
self-stimulated laughter with the wisdom of Eastern health
systems.

There are now an estimated 10,000 Laughter Clubs throughout the world, according to Dr. Kataria. More information can be found at www.laughteryoga.org. Thanks to the participation of several Certified Laughter Yoga Leaders, Laguna Beach has the fame of being the first Laughter Club in the world outside of India to offer the health-building practice seven days per week. Other Laguna Beach residents who regularly lead Laughter Club exercises are David Sullenger, Kathryn Burns, Ruthe Gluckson, David Fleischmann, Linda Morphew and Dorothy Meyers.

Laughter Club Leader Briar claims that "Laughter practices are safe and effective; they require no special equipment or clothing; they increase your sense of humor, improve interpersonal relations, and enhance your enjoyment of life in general". Briar says that Laughter Club members tend to develop caring, fun friendships.

"Laughter is the shortest distance between two people." -- Victor Borge

Laughter Club Founder Jeffrey Briar is a Graduate of The Dr. Kataria School of Laughter Yoga, having completed their Teacher Training program in Switzerland in 2005. One of the leading exponents of this practice in the USA, Briar recently became the Director of The Laughter Yoga Institute. Mr. Briar regularly gives Trainings for new Laughter Yoga leaders. He is also a Yoga teacher of 40 years' experience, and a former professional comedian and character actor who has worked with Bruce Willis, Blake Edwards, Steven Spielberg, Mariel Hemingway and many others. Mr. Briar leads the Laguna Laughter Club as a free public service. He also offers Laughter Yoga classes, workshops and seminars, and corporate stress-reduction programs.

Laguna Laughter Club meetings are suitable for all ages and levels of ability, and everyone is welcome to join them on the beach in Laguna. For more information, call (949) 376-1939, email JBriar@LYInstitute.org, or visit their website at www.JoyfulB.com.

-end-

PLEASE RUN THROUGH (date)

CLYL LEADER TRAINING SCHEDULE: Day 1

(as suggested by the Dr. Kataria School Teacher's Manual; revised by Jeffrey Briar 2011)

Two days, 8-hours daily (with 1-hour lunch break)

Time	Workshop Details
8:30	Completion of Registration Forms & Liability Release
9:00 – 9.10	Introduction of CLY Teacher (self). Venue logistics, rest rooms, lunch and tea/coffee places, timings of the breaks and rules for the venue, etc.
9:10 – 9.30	Video clips: International news coverage. Complete 'How do you feel?' form.
9:30 – 10.00	Participant Introductions: Group exercise seated in a tight circle. Members tell their name, where they live, and their job -- laughing after each statement. Group dialogue – what did we learn from this exercise?
10:00 – 11.00	Laughter Yoga, history, Teacher's story, concept, philosophy with warm up exercises spaced between and laughter/playfulness to break the monotony.
11:00 – 11.20	Tea/Coffee Break
11:20 – 12.30	Laughter Yoga session (10 Foundation Exercises). Teacher presents and demonstrates with student participation. Laughter Meditation followed by Guided Relaxation.
12:30 – 1:30	LUNCH
1:30 – 3.00	Laughter Yoga Leader basic facilitation skills: 4 steps of Laughter Yoga. Introduction then practice of a-c by each participant: a) Clapping – explain acupressure clapping b) Breathing – chanting c) Child-like playfulness – movement & eye contact d) L.Y. Exercises
3:00 – 3.20	Tea/Coffee Break
4:20 – 4.00	Laughter Yoga session (10 more Foundation Exercises). Teacher presents and demonstrates with student participation.
4:00 – 4.30	A quick description: what is Laughter Yoga? (Teacher presentation and demonstration, then student practice).
4:30 – 5.00	Laughter Meditation basics followed by Guided Relaxation – led by the Teacher. Complete side 2 of 'How do you feel?' form and hand in to Teacher.

CLYL LEADER TRAINING SCHEDULE: Day 2

Time	Workshop Details
9:00 – 9.15	Feedback from Day 1: "How did you feel about yesterday?"
9:15 – 9.45	Benefits of Laughter Yoga, scientific research and contra-indications.
9:45 – 11.00	Practice session to continue both practical and theory. Participants practice leading laughter exercises.
11:00 – 11.30	Laughter Yoga in companies and corporations.
11:30 – 12.00	Laughter Yoga session (10 more Foundation Exercises). Teacher presents and demonstrates with student participation. Laughter Meditation followed by Guided Relaxation.
12.00 – 12.30	How to laugh alone. Adding more laughter your life, laughing in the face of challenges. Identifying your stressors and developing laughter exercises for them.
12:30 – 1:30	LUNCH
1:30 – 2.00	Laughter Yoga with seniors – techniques and practice.
2:00 – 3.00	How to start a Laughter Club. Basic guidelines for organizing public seminars, promoting and running Laughter Yoga sessions, media and publicity.
3:00 – 3.30	Laughter Yoga with school children.
3:30 – 4.00	Tea Break.
4:00 – 4.30	Laughter Yoga session (10 more Foundation Exercises) teacher presents and demonstrates with student participation.
4:30 – 5.00	Certification, group photo and networking.

Please note: in 2018, the Leader Training is scheduled to be redesigned with emphasis on: learning to lead Laughter Exercises, and starting/ operating social Laugher Clubs. The specialized communities of Elders, Schoolchildren, and Businesses, along with Healthcare, will be addressed (on an introductory level) in a separate 3rd Day training program. Please stay in contact with The Laughter Yoga Institute and Laughter Yoga International for revised training agendas.

Sample Agenda:
2-Day Certified Laughter Yoga Leader Training
(Alternative Structure from Jeffrey Briar)

ith this structure a person can attend Day One only and they will learn how to lead laughter exercises, along with a basic education in Laughter Yoga history and theory. If they do not attend Day Two they would not learn about: forming a club, working with seniors/schoolkids/businesses, nor giving workshops or otherwise "putting it out into the world". They would not be eligible to receive a diploma nor certification as a "Laughter Yoga Leader" - but they'd make a great Laughter Club *helper*!

DAY ONE: Mastering Laughter Leadership
"Getting It *In ♥ Here*" (in the heart)

Sign In. Background. Ground/Venue rules.

- **Introductions with laughing ("My name is... I am from... What I do is...").**

Laughing for No Reason. Discussion : what we learned from that exercise (we can laugh when we choose to; felt energetic, friendly, etc.)

- Theory. "Feeling Good" not needed. Neutralizing the judgmental mind

The joyful nature of humanity and Contagiousness of Laughter. Q's and A's.

* **Warming Up** the Voice
* History of Laughter Yoga, Therapy, Clubs. Clapping. Gibberish Talk I. Yoga Breath I

Definition of Laughter Club = **a group of people who gather together to practice laughter as a form of exercise, cultivating childlike playfulness.**

- Unique features of Laughter Therapy: NOT dependent on jokes. It IS body based, child-like.

1) Don't need a Sense of Humor;   2) Don't need to Feel Good or Be Happy;   3) Don't need any Reason in order to laugh.

DAY ONE, continued

* Distinction between *Happiness* (Conditional: achieving desires/wants) -and- *Joyfulness* (Unconditional: a state of Being, a Choice)
* Practicum : **Laughter Session**   Point out the standard sequence Formula:
1) Laughter practice
2) "Ho, Ho, Ha-ha-ha" Neuro-Linguistic Programming technique ("Motion creates Emotion" – anchoring)
3) Breathing/Stretching practice
Laughter Exercise 3 Types:
1. Based on Yoga postures/breathing;   2. Value-Added (re-program stressful situations);   3. Playful and Acting Games.

Laughter Exercises

Laughter Meditation I.: 1) Sit, eyes open. 2) Lie down, eyes closed.

------

* Instructional Techniques:
1) "Ho ho, ha-ha-ha" with clapping (NLP technique)
2) Yogic Deep Breathing
3) Gibberish talk
4) Practicum: **Laughter Exercises**
 Positive Affirmations

------

* Leadership Coaching: Grounding in case of Overstimulation
Time Scheduling. Restrictions (contraindications, verbalization, distractions). Problem-solving.
*   Practicum: **Laughter Exercises III.** Small **Group Practice**
* Individual Concerns, Testimonials
* Sign Out

DAY TWO: Sharing the Chemistry of Happiness
"Putting It *Out There*" (into the world)

Sign In
Conversational **Gibberish**
* **"The Inner Spirit of Laughter, and The Meaning of Life."**
  Art and Science of Gibberish. Catharsis of emotions ("We are
  meaning-making machines").
* Practicum: **Gibberish Meditation and Progressive Relaxation**

------

* Applications of cathartic gibberish.
1) If can't do Laughter Meditation
2) As part of Solo Practice: 5 min. gibberish, then lie down → leads
   to Spontaneous Laughter * Effect of gibberish is DEEPEST *WITH
   EYES CLOSED* * (and big, expressive physical movement)
* **Review**: To Laugh, You need: No Jokes, No Sense of Humor, No
  Reason
  →**Presentations to the Press** as a Laughter Yoga Leader
Why the word, "Yoga"? Combined breathing exercises from Yoga,
   changes mind (relaxation, peace, happiness)
A Laughter Club = people gather together, cultivate playfulness,
   willingness to laugh (for no reason: no jokes required)
* **Presenting to Media.** Personal story
Giving seminars (physical requests)
* **Laughter Exercises**

------

* ***Solo Practice*** Make it a habit in 40 days
* **Starting a Laughter Club**. Non-political, non-religious. Free (at
  cost). Objective = to bring Health, Joyfulness, and World Peace.
Core group. Awareness and Promotion. Members' creative
  participation. Value Additions; networking/socializing.
  Applications.
* **Laughter Exercises**

------

* Special-Needs Groups:

1. *Seniors* (Disclaimer, Staff Member in case of emergency); Liability Insurance

2. *Corporate/Business World* Legitimacy/scientific data

Scientifically Proven TO REDUCE STRESS in the workplace --- Economical -- Easy to learn -- Easy to practice. Most economical; least time consuming. Reduce Absenteeism, Create Positive Work Environment. Builds Teamwork and Partnership. Cost-effective.

Other **Income-producing events**: Laughter Bus, Gibberish Party, Cruise, Laughter/Creativity/Dance Workshop/Party, Laughter Yoga Holiday, Retreat, for Couples ("Connection not correction"), Specialized Workshops. **Brainstorming**.

Laughter Exercise Session (with new Leaders guiding an exercise)

BREAK (Prepare for Graduation)

* Special-Needs Groups

3. *Children*: "Follow the Leader," trade off

Questions and Answers. Concerns and Acknowledgements
    Graduation Ceremony, Presentation of Diplomas
Group Photograph; Sign Out

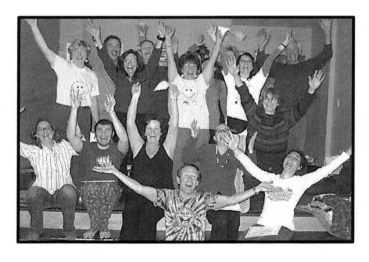

CHECKLIST FOR THE TWO-DAY CERTIFIED LAUGHTER YOGA LEADER TRAINING

Edited and Revised by Jeffrey Briar

Day One:

o Completion of Registration Forms
o Completion of Liability Release
o Introduction of the Certified Laughter Yoga Teacher (Teacher's experience)
o Venue Logistics (restrooms, lunch and tea breaks, timings of the breaks, venue rules, etc.)
o Video Clips: International News Coverage
o "How Do You Feel?" Form (Side One)
o Participant Introductions, as a Group Exercise: in a tight circle, members say 1. Their name, 2. Where they live, and 3. What they do for a living (or something they like to do: a hobby or pastime), laughing after each statement. After each participant concludes, all say: "Very good, very good, Yay!"
o Group Dialogue – What did we learn from that exercise?
  We can laugh for no reason
  Improved mood
  Feel refreshed, more energetic

Less pain

Feel more connected and friendly toward others

Things which might have been stressful (introducing oneself to strangers) can be stress-free

o History of Laughter Yoga

Dr. Kataria writing article "Laughter the Best Medicine"

Idea of Laughter Club – asked 200 people

Began with 5 people in a park in Mumbai (soon grew to 50) – at first used jokes

Ran out of jokes, or jokes proved offensive or ineffective

Theory of Motion creates Emotion

Laughed more without jokes than the previous two weeks using jokes (thanks to eye contact and interpersonal playfulness)

o Teacher's Personal Story
o Laughter Yoga Concept and Philosophy (with warm-up exercises interspersed between laughter/playfulness to break the monotony)
o Laughter Yoga Session (10 foundation exercises): Teacher presents and demonstrates with student participation

o Laughter Meditation
   Seated, eyes open ; and
   Lying down, eyes closed
o Guided Relaxation
o Complete Side Two of "How Do You Feel?" Form
o Laughter Yoga Leader Basic Facilitation Skills:
   Four Steps of Laughter Exercise Session
   1. Clapping and Warming-up Exercises -- explain acupressure clapping ("Ho, ho, ha-ha-ha")
   2. Deep Breathing Exercises -- stretching, chanting, slap thighs and run around
   3. Childlike Playfulness -- movement and eye contact ("Very good, very good, Yay!")
   4. Laughter Exercises -- yogic; physical/playful; value-based
o Each Participant Practices Steps 1 through 3
o Laughter Yoga Session (10 more foundation exercises): Teacher presents and demonstrates with student participation.
o Includes Laughter Meditation, and
o Guided Relaxation
o A quick description "What is Laughter Yoga?" (Teacher presentation and demonstration, then student practice)
o Laughter Meditation Basics
o Guided Relaxation -- led by the teacher

NOTES:
> Twenty Laughter Exercises experienced (minimum).

RECOMMENDED on Day One:
- Gibberish 1 as a warm-up to get into Playfulness
- **Five Points: "What is Laughter Yoga?"**

....

Day Two:

o Feedback from Day 1 – How did you feel about yesterday?
o Benefits of Laughter Yoga (Scientific Research and Contraindications)
o Practice Session (to continue practical and theory): Participants practice leading exercises
o **[Laughter Yoga in Companies and Corporations]**
o Laughter Yoga Session (10 more foundation exercises): Teacher presents and demonstrates with student participation
o Includes Laughter Meditation and
o Guided Relaxation
o How to Laugh Alone – Adding more laughter to your life, laughing in the face of challenges,

identifying personal stressors and developing laughter exercises for them, etc.
- o [**Laughter Yoga With Seniors** – techniques and practice]
- o How to Start a Laughter Club – Basic guidelines for organizing public seminars, promoting and running Laughter Yoga Sessions, media and publicity
- o [**Laughter Yoga With School Children**]
- o Laughter Yoga Session (10 more foundation exercises): Teacher presents and demonstrates with student participation
- o Certification, Group Photo(s), Networking

NOTES:
- ➤ Twenty Laughter Exercises experienced today (40 minimum over the two days).
- ➤ Each student has had experience leading at least one Laughter Exercise (supervised by a certified Teacher).

....

RECOMMENDED at some point during the two days:

- Each participant introduces themself to the group (experience, vision of what they want to do with laughter)

- **Three Reasons: "Why do Laughter Yoga / Why go to a Laughter Club?"**
- Practice giving a basic presentation to media (radio interviewer)
- Multiple experiences of students leading Laughter Exercises
- Gibberish 2 for cathartic emotional release.
- "Ha Ha" Mantra (Life's Little Stresses/Free-Floating Hostilities - Compassionate Laughter)
- Dr. Kataria's life story (before Laughter Yoga: villager, actor, doctor, explorer, Man of Action)
- "Ho, ho, ha, ha Grounding Dance" (audio)

Laughter Yoga Philosophy to include

o Distinction between *Happiness* (depends on conditions being satisfied) and *Joyfulness* (unconditional).

o *The Meaning of Life* : Life itself is meaningless; human beings automatically make things mean something; we can choose what we make things mean. Life is a joke and "The sense of humor of God is weird." (- Dr. Kataria) o *The Inner Spirit of Laughter* : We laugh not just for ourselves, but to bring joy to others and the world. Joy is our nature; it is always available as a choice to tap into.

Leader Trainees are to receive:
✓ Leader Training Manual (Teacher's option whether as digital files, as hardcopy on paper, or both)
✓ Certificate (diploma) which Teacher obtains from headquarters, bearing the signatures of Dr. Kataria (facsimile) and the certified Teacher
✓ Practice leading laughter exercise(s) while being supervised/coached by the Teacher and/or another qualified Laughter Yoga professional

(Please see note on the bottom of p. 106 regarding Leader Trainings in 2018 and beyond)

Based on the work and teachings of Dr. Madan Kataria
www.laughteryoga.org
Edited and Revised by Jeffrey Briar
The Laughter Yoga Institute :: www.LYInstitute.org
790 Manzanita Dr. Laguna Beach, California 92651-1962 USA
(949) 376-1939   Jeffrey@laughteryoga.org

Files available on the **Laugh4Health** Yahoogroup **website** http://health.groups.yahoo.com/group/Laugh4Health

Several hundred documents are available, downloadable at no charge. Sample topics:

- Foundation Exercises
- Hundreds more Laughter Exercises, in several languages
- Marketing Ideas
- Workshop Agendas : Yoga classes, Laughter Cruises, Retreats
- Banner Design
- Proposals (Corporate, Yoga Studios, many more)
- Sample Contracts
- Games
- Presentations (at Conferences, on various topics)
- Flyers (Club Sessions, Parties, Special Events, many more)
- Gibberish Specialty Items
- Meditations
- Insurance Resources
- Laughter in the Brain
- Letter of Recommendation (model)
- Script for Laughter Club Entry in a Parade
- Song Lyrics

"Very good, very good, Yay!"
in many languages

Afrikaans : Baie Goed, Baie Goed, Yey!

Arabic : Waajid Zain..Waajid Zain, Yeahhh

Armenian : Shad lav, shad lav or bagus, bagus yay!

Bengali : Khoob Bhalo, Khoob Bhalo, Yay!

Burmese : Ree Doo Mah, Ree Doo Mah, EAYYY!

Chinese : Fei-chang-hau, fei-chang-hau, yay!

Croatian : Dobro je, dobro je, jeeeeeej!

Danish : Rigtig dejlig, rigtig dejlig, aar!

Dutch : Heel goed , heel goed, Ja!

English : Very Good, Very Good, Yay! (British :
    "Jolly Good, Jolly Good, Huzzah!")

Filipino : Magaling Magaling Magaling! Wuhoooooo!
Wootwoot!

Finnish : Tosi hyvä, tosi hyvä, jee!"

French : Tres Bien, Tres bien, Ouai! Or C'est super,
    C'est super; or C'est superbe, c'est superbe!

Gaelic : Gle mhah, gle mhah, yay!

German : Sehr gut, sehr gut – Jah!

Gujerati : ketlu saaroo, ketlu saroo, Yey!

Hebrew : Tov Meod, Tov Meod, Yesh!

Hindi : Bahut acchaa , Bahut acchaa , yeeeeeee!
    Also Hindi: Bahot badhiya, Bahot badhiya, Yey!

Hungarian : Jaj de jo, Jaj de jo, Hurra!!!!

Indonesia : Bagus..bagus sekali, yaaayyy!

Italian : Molto bene, molto bene, yeah!

"Very good, very good, Yay!" in different languages

Japanese : Yattah, yattah, Yeah!

Kannada : Chanagide, Chanagide, Yay!

Lithuanian : Labai gerai, labai gerai, jeeee!

Malay: Bagus! Bagus! Yee-eaah!

Malayalam : Valare Nallathu.. Valare Nallathu..
    Yeah….

Marathi : Khoob Chaan, Khoob Chaan, Yay!
    Also Marathi: Lay Bhari, Lay Bhari, Yay!

Norwegian : Veldig Bra, Veldig Bra, Yay!

Polish : Bardzo dobrze, bardzo dobrze, Yay!

Portuguese : Muito Bom, Muito Bom, Sim!

Punjabi : Vadda Changa, Vadda Changa, Yay!

Romanian : Foarte Bine, Foarte Bine, Yay!
    (pronounced "fuarte beena")

Russian : … harasho, harasho, yay!

Sindhi : Dado Suttho, Dado Suttho, Yay!

Spanish : Muy bien, muy bien, yeah! (or "…-Orale!")

Sudtyrolian (Sudtirolerisch) : Volle, volle, Guat!

Sweden : Mycket Bra, Mycket Bra, Ja!

Tamil : Rombo Nalla Irukku, Rombo Nalla Irukku,
    Yey! (Or: Nalla Irk, Nalla Irk, Yey!)

Telugu : Chaala Bagundhi, Chaala Bagundhi, He!

Turkish : Hah hah hah Çok?yi Çok?yi, Evet!

Alternative Terms
instead of Laughter "YOGA"

Laughter Class, Program, Retreat, Seminar, Workshop

Laughter Circle
Laughter Exercise
Laughter for Health
Laughter for Life
Laughter for Lungs

Laugh `n Stretch
Laugh Yourself Healthy
Laugh Yourself Well
Laughter Wellness (kudos to Sebastien Gendry)
Laugh for the Health of It
Laughter Workout
Laughter Party
Laugharobics
Laughterobics
Laughilates (Laugh-a-Lot-Ease)

Fun & Laughter
Healthy Stress Management Techniques
Stretch and Laugh
Stress Management
Stress Relief
Stress Relief through Laughter
Therapeutic Laughter

Alternative Terms
Instead of "Fake" Laughter

Deliberate Laughter
Free Laughter
Healthy Laughter (Healthy Laughing)
Intentional Laughter
Laughter-On-Purpose
Pretend Laughter
Pro-active Laughter (vs. "Re-active" Laughter)
Self-Generated Laughter
Self-Induced Laughter
Self-Stimulated Laughter
Simulated Laughter
Strategic Laughter
Unconditional Laughter
Voluntary Laughter
Willful Laughter

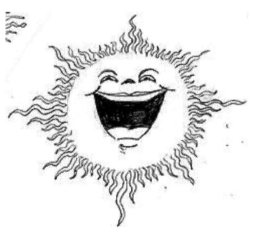

Art by Lynn Kubasek

Making Money with Laughter-Based Programs

By Jeffrey Briar, Director of The Laughter Yoga Institute

Some Ways People are Sharing Laughter Professionally
(getting paid)

1. Consultant to businesses, stores, and corporations. Use laughter to boost employee morale, reduce turnover, relieve stress, encourage teamwork and spark creativity.

2. Yoga-plus: add laughter practices to a traditional Hatha Yoga class, to support good breathing practices and ease tension. Laughter is especially good before Final Relaxation.

3. Laughter Bus: 8 a.m. laugh session. Go to scenic roadside picnic spots, do two or three exercises at each. The bus has an audio system; during the trip, everyone shares about themselves, sings/shares jokes (sometimes in gibberish), etc. Stop for lunch, tea. Bring business cards to share with the fascinated folks who see you at the stops!

4. Chambers of Commerce and other service/business groups (Moose, Lions, Optimists, Rotary, etc.) want speakers for luncheons or meetings; sometimes for pay. This often makes for good connections to other companies that can use a Laughter Leader.

5. Laughter Doctor/Therapist: If you are qualified to call yourself a "Therapist", add Therapeutic Laughter to your specialties.

6. Add laughter for a "Stress Relief Break" for any intense coaching: golf, tennis, other sports; chess tournaments, Sudoku matches, etc.

7. Special Gatherings: Wedding, Bachelor Party, Bar Mitzvah -- be their "Laughter Blaster".

8. Laughter Cruise. Can take place on a luxury liner, or a smaller semi-private ship. Lead sessions, train staff, and/or provide experiential lectures. www.LaughterCruise.com.

9. Yacht Parties.

10. Airlines (On-board Laughter Leader; or train the Hosts/Hostesses).

11. Laughter Tour, Laughter Walk, Laughter Hike: Have a picnic after hike, perhaps with a bonfire. Do singalongs, in gibberish or with all-laughter verses. Offer to guide a trip for the Sierra Club – laughing in the wilds of nature.

12. Laughter Hayrides and Sleigh Rides.

13. Wine Tasting.

14. Icebreaker: Singles Groups, Church Groups. Any "get to know the new folks" gathering.

15. Adult Care Homes, Senior Centers; Hospitals; Cancer Support Groups - virtually *all* Support Groups.

16. Charter Schools (most are required to have Physical Education programs).

17. Prisons.

18. Rehab/Treatment Centers; Abused Women's/Children's Shelters.

19. Laughilates (Laffilates). Mix Laughter with Pilates exercises.

20. SoberVacations.com. Provide happy body chemistry, with no negative side effects!

21. LaughterCam: live, online laughter session.

22. Produce special topic DVD's and other merchandise to help Laughter Leaders.

23. "Laugh For The Cure" - for depression, MS, other maladies.

24. Personal Laughter Coach. One-on-One Laughter Coaching, see videos at www.laughteryoga.org.

25. Laughter Makeover – change your looks as well as your attitude.

26. Stress Relief for Students - help relax, improve test scores.

27. Health and Resort Spas; Gyms.

28. College Teacher: offer classes through Physical Education Department. Don't forget Senior/Emeritus/Lifelong Learning Programs. Also Psychology, Social Sciences, Health departments.

29. Family Night at Dance Studios – have the students bring siblings, boyfriends, schoolmates, parents, grandparents.

30. College Re-entry Programs, Single Parents' Support Groups, Stress-Management Classes.

31. Laughter Club Tours: Travel to different Laughter Clubs to network, learn, and share friendship.

32. What do you LOVE to do? Do it with Laughter -and Laughter Buddies!

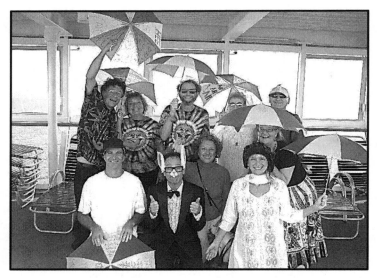

Scene from a Laughter Cruise

Sample Contract

THE LAUGHTER YOGA INSTITUTE

790 Manzanita Dr.
Laguna Beach, CA 92651-1962
info@LYInstitute.org   www.LYInstitute.org

Agreement:

Ordered by (Host):   Rxxxxx Txxx, B. S.
Executive Event Planner | MajorOrg Inc.
4141 Main Street, Plantain, Washington 10019-0065
Phone: (xxx) XXX-XXXX
Email: RaxxyTaxxy@majorg.com

Service:
The Laughter Yoga Institute
agrees to provide a trained Instructor for an
experiential program entitled:

"Laughter Yoga - A Breakthrough Health Technology"

for a group of approximately 250 persons

Friday, November xx, 20XX, 6:15-7:30pm,
Ambassador Ballroom, Excelsior Hotel, 1100 Excellent
Road, Newcastle Beach California 92469
For a fee of $350 (three hundred fifty dollars exactly).
Host will provide: appropriate stage lighting,
microphone and sound amplification.

Payment Terms:
A check for the honorarium fee of $350 (Three
Hundred Fifty Dollars Exactly) will be mailed promptly

following the service date to The Laughter Yoga Institute at the address provided at the top of this page.

The Laughter Yoga Institute uses FEIN # XX-XXXXXXX.

Agreed,

Jerfej Ebiarb

._____.   ._____.
Jeffrey Briar, Director   Date
The Laughter Yoga Institute

._____.   ._____.
For MajorOrg Inc.   Date

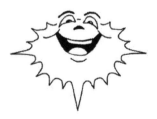

At The Laughter Yoga Institute, We Take Laughter Seriously.

Articles/Books on Laughter (and Humor)
(Also see "Resources" p. 15X)

The following list was compiled by Don L. F. Nilsen, English Department, Arizona State University Tempe, AZ, with a few additions by Jeffrey Briar and others. Find more at www.BioMedSearch.com and via www.laughterremedy.com.

Adelswärd, Viveka, and Britt-Marie Öberg. "The Function of Laughter and Joking in Negotiating Activities." HUMOR: International Journal of Humor Research 11.4 (1998): 411-430.

Arner, T. D. "No Joke: Transcendent Laughter in The Teseida and The Miller's Tale." Studies in Philology 102.2 (2005).

Askenasy, J. J. M. "The Functions and Dysfunctions of Laughter." Journal of General Psychology 14.4 (1987): 317-34.

Bainy, Moses. Why Do We Laugh and Cry? West Ryde, Australia: Sunlight Publications, 1993.

Basil Hall, Laughter as a displacement activity: the implications for humor theory

Baudelaire, Charles. The Essence of Laughter. New York, NY: Meridian: 1956.

Bell, N. D. "Laughter in Interaction." Discourse Studies 7.1 (2005): 137-138.

Bellert, J. "Humor: A Therapeutic Approach in Oncology Nursing." Cancer Nursing 12.2 (1989): 65-70.

Berger, Arthur Asa. "After the Laughter: A Concluding Note." Blind Men and Elephants: Perspectives on Humor. New Brunswick, NJ: Transaction Press, 1995, 159-170.

Berger, Arthur Asa. "The Functions of Laughter: Sociological Aspects of Humor." Blind Men and Elephants: Perspectives on Humor. New Brunswick, NJ: Transaction Press, 1995, 91-104.

Berger, Arthur Asa. "The Politics of Laughter: A Cultural Theory of Humor Preferences." Blind Men and Elephants: Perspectives on Humor. New Brunswick, NJ: Transaction Press, 1995, 105-120.

Berger, Arthur Asa. "The Problem of Laughter: Philosophical Approaches to Humor." Blind Men and Elephants: Perspectives on Humor. New Brunswick, NJ: Transaction Press, 1995, 37-50.

Berger, Arthur Asa. Redeeming Laughter. New York, NY: Walter de Gruyter, 1997.

Berger, Arthur Asa. "The Rhetoric of Laughter: The Techniques Used in Humor." Blind Men and Elephants: Perspectives on Humor. New Brunswick, NJ: Transaction Press, 1995, 51-64.

Berger, Arthur Asa. "Seeing Laughter: Visual Aspects of Humor." Blind Men and Elephants: Perspectives on Humor. New Brunswick, NJ: Transaction Press, 1995, 139-158.

Berger, Arthur Asa. "The Structure of Laughter: Semiotics and Humor." Blind Men and Elephants: Perspectives on Humor. New Brunswick, NJ: Transaction Press, 1995, 65-78.

Berger, Arthur Asa, and A. Wildavsky. "Who Laughs at What?" Society 31.6 (1994): 82-86.

Berger, Peter L. Redeeming Laughter: The Comic Dimension of Human Experience. Hawthorne, NY: Walter de Gruyter, 1997.

Berger, Phil. The Last Laugh. NY: Limelight, 1985.

Bergler, E. Laughter and the Sense of Humor. NY: Intercontinental Medical Book Corp, 1956.

Bergson, Henri Louis. Laughter: An Essay on the Meaning of the Comic. New York, NY: MacMillan, 1924.

Bergson, Henri Louis. "Laughter." Comedy. Ed. Wylie Sypher. Garden City, NY: Doubleday, 1956, 59-190.

Berk, Lee, and S. A. Tan. "Eustress of Mirthful Laughter Modulates the Immune System Lymphokine Interferon-Gama." Annals of Behavioral Medicine Supplement, Proceedings of the Society of Behavioral Medicine's Sixteenth Annual Scientific Sessions 17 (1995): C064.

Berk, Lee, S. A. Tan, and William Fry. "Eustress of Humor Associated Laughter Modulates Specific Immune System Components." Annals of Behavioral Medicine Supplement, Proceedings of the Society of Behavioral Medicine's Fourteenth Annual Scientific Sessions 15 S111.

Berk, Lee., S. A. Tan, William F. Fry, B. J. Napier, J. W. Lee, R. W. Hubbard, J. E. Lewis, and W. C. Eby. "Neuroendrocrine and Stress Hormone Changes During Mirthful Laughter." American Journal of the Medical Sciences. 298.6 (1989): 390-96.

Berk, Lee, S. Tan, B. Napier, and W. Evy. "Eustress of Mirthful Laughter Modifies Natural Killer Cell Activity. Clinical Research 37 (1989): 115A.

Berk, Lee, S. A. Tan, S. Nehlsen-Cannarella, B. J. Napier, J. E. Lewis, J. E. Lee, and W. C. Eby. "Humor Associated with Laughter Decreases Cortisol and Increases Spontaneous Lymphocyte Blastogenesis." Clinical Research 36 (1988): 435A.

Berlyne, D. E. "Laughter, Humor, and Play." Handbook of Social Psychology: Volume 3. Eds. G. Lindzey, and E. Aronson. Reading, MA: Addison-Wesley, 1969.

Bizi, S., G. Keinan, and B. Beit-Hallahi. "Humor and Coping with Stress: A Test Under Real-Life conditions." Personality and Individual Differences 9 (1988): 951-956.

Black, D. W. "Laughter." Journal of the American Medical Association 252.21 (1984): 2995-98.

Black, D. W. "Pathological Laughter." Journal of Nervous and Mental Diseases 170 (1982): 67-71.

Blumenfeld, E., and L. Alpern. The Smile Connection: How to Use Humor in Dealing with People. Englewood Cliffs, NJ: Prentice Hall, 1986.

Bonaiuto, Marino, Elio Castellana, and Antonio Pierro. "Arguing and Laughing: The Use of Humor to Negotiate in Group Discussions." HUMOR: International Journal of Humor Research 16.2 (2003): 183-224.

Bornstein, M. H., and M. E. Arterberry. "Recognition, Discrimination and Categorization ofSmiling by 5-Month-Old Infants." Developmental Science 6.5 (2003): 585-599.

Boston, Richard. An Anatomy of Laughter. London, England: Collins, 1974.

Bouissac, Paul. "A Laughable Theory of Laughter." High Quality 22 (1992): 8-11.

Boyd, B. "Laughter and Literature: A Play Theory of Humor." Philosophy and Literature 28.1 (2004): 1-22.

Braga, S. S., R. Manni, and R. F. Pedretti. "Laughter-Induced Syncope." Lancet (July 30-August 6, 2005): 366-426.

Brody, R. "Anatomy of a Laugh." American Health. (Dec, 1983): 43-47.

Briar, Jeffrey. The Great Big Anthology of Laughter Exercises. Laguna Beach, California: Creative Arts Press, 2011.

Briar, Jeffrey. Laughter Revolutionaries, Making the World Safe for Hilarity. Laguna Beach, California: Creative Arts Press, 2011.

Briar, Jeffrey. The Laughter Yoga Book. Laguna Beach, California: Creative Arts Press, 2016.

Brottman, Mikita. "Risus Sardonicus: Neurotic and Pathological Laughter." HUMOR: International Journal of Humor Research. 15.4 (2002): 401-418.

Brown, G. E., D. Brown, and J. Ramos. "Effects of a Laughing Versus a Non-Laughing Model on Humor: Responses in College Students." Psychological Relports 48.1 (1981): 35-40.

Brown, G. E., K. J. Wheeler, and M. Cash. "The Effects of a Laughing vs. a Non-laughing Model on Humor Responses in Preschool Children." Journal of Experimental Child Psychology 29 (1980): 334-39.

Buckley, Francis H. The Morality of Laughter. Ann Arbor, MI: University of Michigan Press, 2003.

Burns, David D. Feeling Good Handbook, The. New York, NY Plume/Penguin, 1999.

Bushnell, D. D., and T. J. Scheff. "The Cathartic Effects of Laughter on Audiences." The Study of Humor. Eds. Harvey Mindess and Joy Turek. Los Angeles, CA: Antioch Univ, 1979, 62ff.

Caron, James E. "From Ethology to Aesthetics: Evolution as a Theoretical Paradigm for Research on Laughter, Humor, and Other Comic Phenomena." HUMOR: International Journal of Humor Research 15.3 (2002): 245-282.

Carroll, Noel. "Words, Images, and Laughter." Persistence of Vision 14 (1997): 42-52.

Casadonte, Donald. "A Note on the Neuro-Mathematics of Laughter." HUMOR: International Journal of Humor Research 16.2 (2003): 133-156.

Chapman, Antony J. "Humor and Laughter in Social Interaction and Some Implications. Handbook of Humor Research, Volume I. Eds. P. E. McGhee, and J. H. Goldstein. New York, NY: Springer, 1983, 135-157.

Chapman, Antony J. "Social Facilitation of Laughter in Children." Journal of Experimental Social Psychology 9 (1973): 528-41.

Chapman, Antony J., and W. Chapman. "Responsiveness to Humor: Its Dependency upon a Companion's Humorous Smiling and Laughter." The Journal of Psychology 88 (1974): 245-52.

Chapman, Antony J., and Hugh C. Foot, eds. Humor and Laughter: Theory, Research, and Applications. New Brunswick, NJ: Transaction, 1996.

Chapman, Antony J., and D. S. Wright. "Social Enhancement of Laughter: An Experimental Analysis of Some Companion Variables." Journal of Experimental Child Psychology 21 (1976).

Charland, M. "Normes and Laughter in Rhetorical Culture." Quarterly Journal of Speech 80.3 (1994): 339-342.

Chase, Jefferson S. Inciting Laughter: The Development of "Jewish Humor" in 19th Century German Culture. New York, NY: Walter de Gruyter, 1999.

Claassens, L. J. M. "Laughter and Tears: Carnivalistic Overtones in the Stories of Sarah and Hagar." Perspectives in Religious Studies 32.3 (2005): 295-308.

Cleveland, Les. Dark Laughter: War in Song and Popular Culture. Westport, CT: Greenwood, 1994.

Cogan, R., D. Cogan, W. Waltz, and M. McCue. "Effects of Laughter and Relaxation on Discomfort Thresholds." Journal of Behavioral Medicine. 10.2 (1987): 139-144.

Coser, R. L. "Laughter among Colleagues." Psychiatry 23 (1960): 81-95.

Coser, R. L. "Some Social Functions of Laughter: A Study of Humor in a Hospital Setting." Human Relations 12.2 (1959).

Cousins, Norman. "The Laughter Prescription." The Saturday Evening Post Oct, 1990: 34.

Cousins, Norman. "Proving the Power of Laughter." Psychology Today 23 (1989: 22-25.

Cox, Samuel S. Why We Laugh. New York: Benjamin Blom, 1969.

Dardick, G. "Learning to Laugh on the Job Principal 69.5 (1990): 32, 34.

Darwin, Charles. "Joy, High Spirits, Love, Tender Feelings, Devotion." The Expression of Emotions in Man and Animals. New York, NY: D. Appleton, 1924, 196-219.

Davidhizar, Ruth, and Margaret Bowen. "The Dynamics of Laughter." Archives of Psychiatric Nursing. 6.2 (1992): 132-137.

Davidson, Cathy N. "Laughter without Comedy in For Whom the Bell Tolls." Hemingway Notes 3.2 (1973): 609

Davis, Jessica Milner. "Taking Humour and Laughter Seriously." Australian Journal of Comedy. 2.1 (1996): 77-88.

de Sousa, Ronald. "When Is It Wrong to Laugh?" The Philosophy of Laughter and Humor. Ed. John Morreall. Albany, NY: State University of New York Press, 1987, 226-249.

Debenham, Warren. Laughter on Record: A Comedy Discography. Metuchen, NJ: The Scarecrow Press, 1988.

Delahaye, S. "Death by Laughter in Sade and Maupassant." French Studies Bulletin 96 (2005): 16-17.

Derks, Peter, Lynn S. Gillikin, Debbie S. Bartolome-Rull, and Edward H. Bogart. "Laughter and Electroencephalographic

Activity." HUMOR: International Journal of Humor Research 10.3 (1997): 285-300.

Devereux, Paul G., and Gerald P. Ginsburg. "Sociality Effects on the Production of Laughter." Journal of General Psychology "Special Issue on Humor and Laughter" Eds. Mahony, Diana L. and Louis G. Lippman.128.2 (2001): 227-240.

Dickie, S. "Joseph Andrews and the Great Laughter Debate." Studies in Eighteenth Century Culture 34 (2005): 271-332.

Dillon, K., B. Minchoff, and K. Baker. "Positive Emotional States and Enhancement of the Immune System." International Journal of Psychiatric Medicine 15 (1985): 13-18.

Ding, G. F., and A. T. Jersild. "A Study of the Laughing and Smiling of Preschool Children." Journal of Genetic Psychology 40 (1932): 452-472.

Dixon, N. "Humor: A Cognitive Alternative to Stress?" Stress and Anxiety. Eds. I. Sarason and C. Spielberger. 7 (1980): 281-289.

Dobbin, J. Individual Differences in th Appraisal of Stress and the Immunological Consequences: Psychological Moderation of Lymphocyte Activation and Cytokine Production. Ontario, Canada: University of Western Ontario, 1990.

Donoghu, E. E., M. W. McCarrey, and R. Clement. "Humor Appreciation as a Function of Canned Laughter, A Mirthful Companion, and Field Dependence–Facilation and Inhibitory Effects." Canadian Journal of Behavioural Science 15.2 (1983).

Doskoch, P. "Happily ever Laughter." Psychology Today July/August, 1996): 33-35.

Dossey, L. "Now You Are Fit to Live: Humor and Health." Alternative Therapies 2.5 (1996): 8-13, 98-100.

Dudden, Arthur P. The Assault of Laughter. New York, NY: A. S. Barnes, 1962.

Dvorakova, Alena. "Laughing at Nothing: Humor as a Response to Nihilism." British Journal of Aesthetics 45.1 (2005): 106-108.

Eastman, Max. Enjoyment of Laughter. NY: Simon and Schuster, 1936.

Eckardt, A. Roy. Sitting in the Earth and Laughing: A Handbook of Humor. New Brunswick, NJ: Transaction, 1992.

Elliot-Binns, C. P. "Laughter and Medicine." Journal of the Royal Coll Gen Pract 35.8 (1985): 364-65.

Elsley, Judy. "Laughter as Feminine Power in The Color Purple and A Question of Silence." New Perspectives on Women and

Comedy. Ed. Regina Barreca. Philadelphia, PA: Gordon and Breach, 1992, 193-200.

Erdman, L. "Laughter Therapy for Patients with Cancer." Oncology Nursing Forum 18.8 (1991): 1359-1363.

Falk, Dana R., and Clara E. Hill. "Counselor Interventions Preceding Client Laughter in Brief Therapy." Journal of Counseling Psychology 39.1 (1992): 39-45.

Farley-Hills, David. The Benevolence of Laughter: Comic Poetry of the Commonwealth and Restoration. Totowa, NJ: Rowman and Littlefield, 1974.

Fendt, G. "Apartheid among the Dead; Or, on Christian Laughter in Ann Petry's `The Bones of Louella Brown.'" Contributions in AfroAmerican and African Studies 209 (2004).

Finnigan, Jon. Laughing All the Way Home: Indigenous Humour of the Ottawa Valley. Toronto, Canada: Deneau, 1984.

Flewelling, Ralph Tyler. "The Animal Capable of Laughter." Personalist 25 (1944): 341-353.

Flugel, J. C. "Humor and Laughter." Handbook of Social Psychology. Ed. Lindzey. Reading, MA: Addison-Wesley, 1954, 709-34.

Fogarasi, A., J. Janszky, Z. Siegler, and I. Tuxhorn. "Ictal Smile Lateralizes to the Right Hemisphere in Childhood Epilepsy." Epilepsia 46.3 (2005): 449-451.

Foot, Hugh. "Humor and Laughter." A Handbook of Communication Skills. Ed. O. D. W. Hargie. London, England: Croom Helm, 1986, 355-382.

Fox, Kathleen. "Laugh it Off: The Effect of Humor on the Well-Being of the Older Adult." Journal of Gerontological Nursing 16.12 (December, 1990): 11-16.

Francis, L. E. "Laughter: The Best Mediation–Humor as Emotion Management Interaction." Symbolic Interaction 17.2 (1994): 147-163.

Frank, Mark G., and Paul Ekman. "Not all Smiles are Created Equal: The Differences between Enjoyment and Nonenjoyment Smiles." HUMOR: International Journal of Humor Research 6.1 (1993): 6-26.

Fridlund, Alan J. "Sociality of Solitary Smiling: Potentiation by an Implicit Audience." Journal of Personality and Social Psychology. 60 (1991): 229-240.

Fridlund, Alan J., and Jennifer M. Loftis. "Relations between Tickling and Humorous Laughter: Preliminary Support for the Darwin-Hecker Hypothesis." Biological Psychology 30.2 (1990).

Fry, William F. "Laughter: Is It the Best Medicine?" Stanford MD 10.1 (1971): 16-20.

Fry, W. F. and Allan, M. Make 'em Laugh. Palo Alto, CA: Science and Behavior Books, 1975

Fry, William F. "The Respiratory Components of Mirthful Laughter." Journal of Biological Psychology 19.2 (1977): 39-50.

Fry, William F., and William M. Savin. "Mirthful Laughter and Blood Pressure." HUMOR: International Journal of Humor Research 1.1 (1988): 49-62.

Gallo, Nick. "Lighten Up: Laugh Your Way to Good Health." Better Homes and Gardens. August, 1989: 31-32.

Gavioli, Lauri. "Turn-Initial Versus Turn-Final Laughter: Two Techniques for Initiating Remedy in English/Italian Bookshop Service Encounters." Discourse Processes 19 (1995): 369-384.

Gazella, Katie. "Humor at the University of Michigan: A New Study Investigates What Makes Us Laugh, and Why." LSA: College of Literature, Science, and the Arts Magazine (Fall, 2005): 41-42.

Gelbart, Larry. Laughing Matters. New York, NY: Random House, 1998.

Gelkopf, Marc, Shulamith Kreitler, and Mircea Sigal. "Laughter in a Psychiatric Ward: Somatic, Emotional, Social, and Clinical Influences on Schizophrenic Patients." Journal of Nervous and Mental Disease. 185.1 (1993): 283-289.

Gelkopf, Marc, and M. Sigal. "It is Not Enough to Have them Laugh: Hostility, Anger, and Humor-Coping in Schizophrenic Patients." Humor: International Journal of Humor Research 8.3 (1995): 273-284.

Gendry, Sebastien Laughter Works: A Theoretical Framework 2014.

Gervais, Matthew and David Sloane Wilson. "The Evolution of Laughter and Humor: A Synthetic Approach." Quarterly Review of Biology 80.4 (2005): 395-430.

Gierycha, Ewa, Rafal Milnera, and Andrzej Michalskia. "ERP Responses to Smile-Provoking Pictures." Journal of Psychophysiology 19.2 (2005): 77-90.

Giles, H., and G. S. Oxford. "Towards a Multidimensional Theory of Laughter Causation and its Social Implications." Bulletin of the British Psychological Society 23 (1970): 97-105.

Gilligan, B. "A Positive Coping Strategy: Humor in the Oncology Setting." Professional Nurse 8.4 (1993): 231-233.

Gilman, Diane, and Joel Goodman. "Laughing Matters." In Context 13 (Spring, 1986): 11-13.

Glasgow, R. D. V. Madness, Masks, and Laughter. Teaneck, NJ: Farleigh Dickinson University Press, 1995.

Glasgow, R. D. V. Split Down the Sides: On the Subject of Laughter. Lanham, MD: University Press of America, 1997.

Glen, P. "Initiating Shared Laughter in Multi-Party Conversations." Western Journal of Speech Communication 53 (1989): 127-149.

Glenn, Phillip. Laughter in Interaction. Cambridge, England: Cambridge University Press, 2003; reviewed by N. J. Enfield in Linguistics 400 (2005): 1195-1197; reviewed by Salvatore Attardo in HUMOR 18.4 (2005): 422-430.

Goldstein, Jeffrey H. "A Laugh a Day." Sciences 22.6 (1982).

Goldstein, Jeffrey H. "Therapeutic Effects of Laughter." Handbook of Humor and Psychotherapy: Advances in the Clinical Use of Humor. Eds. William Fry and Waleed Salameh. Sarasota, FL: Professional Resource Exchange, 1987, 1-20.

Goodheart, Annette. Laughter Therapy. Santa Barbara, California: Less Stress Press, 1994.

Goodman, Joel. "How to Get More Smileage Out of Your Life: Making Sense of Humor, Then Serving It." Handbook of Research in Humor: Volume 2, Applied Studies Eds. P. E. McGhee, and J. H. Goldstein. New York, NY: Springer-Verlag, 1983, 1-21.

Goodrich, A. J., J. Henry, and D. W. Goodrich. "Laughter in Psychiatric Conferences: A Sociopsychiatric Analysis." American Journal of Orthopsychiatry 24 (1954): 175-184.

Grant, Mary A. The Ancient Rhetorical Theories of the Laughable: The Greek Rhetoricians and Cicero. University of Wisconsin Studies in Language and Literature 21. Madison, WI: University of Wisconsin, 1924.

Gray, Frances. Women and Laughter. Charlottesville, VA: University Press of Virginia, 1994.

Gregory, J. C. The Nature of Laughter. New York, NY: Harcourt, Brace, and Company, 1924.

Greig, J. Y. T. The Psychology of Laughter and Comedy. New York, NY: Cooper Square, 1969.

Grimm, Reinhold, ed. Laughter Unlimited. Seattle, WA: University of Washington Press, 1991.

Gronnerod, J. S. "On the Meanings and Uses of Laughter in Research Interviews: Relationships between Interviewed Men and a Woman Interviewer." Young 12.1 (21004): 31-49.

Gross, E. "Laughter and Symbolic Interaction." Symbolic Interaction 2 (1979): 111-112.

Grotjahn, Martin. "Beyond Laughter: A Summing Up." Comedy: Meaning and Form. Ed. Robert W. Corrigan, San Francisco, CA: Chandler, 1965, 270-276.

Grumet, Gerald W. "Laughter: Nature's Epileptoid Catharsis." Psychological Reports 65 (1989): 1059-1078.

Gruner, Charles R. "Audiences' Response to Jokes in Speeches With and Without, Recorded Laughs." Psychological Reports 73.1 (1993): 347-350.

Gruner, Charles R. The Game of Humor: A Comprehensive Theory of Why We Laugh. New Brunswick, NJ: Transaction, 1997.

Gruner, Charles R. Understanding Laughter: The Workings of Wit and Humor. Chicago: Nelson-Hall, 1978.

Gruner, Charles R., L. J. Pelletier, and M. A. Williams. "Evaluative Responses to Jokes in Informative Speech With and Without Laughter by an Audience: A Partial Replication." Psychological Reports 74 (1994): 446.

Gurevich, Aaron. "Bakhtin and his Theory of Carnival." A Cultural History of Humour: From Antiquity to the Present Day. Eds. Bremmer, Jan, and Herman Roodenburg. Cambridge, England: Polity Press, 1997, 54-60.

Gutwirth, Marcel. Laughing Matter: An Essay on the Comic. Ithaca, NY: Cornell University Press, 1993.

Hageseth, G. A Laughing Place: The Art and Psychology of Positive Humor in Love and Adversity Fort Collins, CO: Berwick, 1988.

Halliwell, S. "Greek Laughter and the Problem of the Absurd." Arion 13.2 (2005): 121-146.

Hanly, Sheila. Peek-A-Boo! 101 Ways to Make a Baby Smile. New York, NY: D. K. Publishers, 1988.

Harral, Stewart. When It's Laughter You're After. Norman, OK: Univ of Oklahoma Press, 1962.

Hawakami, K. K. Takai-Kawakami, M. Tomonaga, J. Suzuki, T. Kusaka, and T. Okay. "Origins of Smiles and Laughter: A Preliminary Study." Early Human Development (2005).

Hayashi, T., O. Urayama, K. Kawai, K. Hayashi, S. Iwanaga, M. Ohta, T. Saito, and K. Murakami. "Laughter Regulates Gene

139

Expression in Patients with Type 2 Diabetes." Psychother.
Psychosom. 75.1 (2006): 62-65.

Hayworth, D. "Social Origin and Function of Laughter."
Psychological Review 35 (1928): 367-384.

Hennenlotter, A., U. Schroeder, P. Erhard, F. Castrop, B.
Haslinger, D. Stoecker, K. W. Lange, and A. O. Caballos-
Bauman. "A Common Neural Basis for Receptive and Expressive
Communicatoin of Pleasant Facial Affect." Neuroimage 26.2
(2005): 581-591.

Herth, K. "Laughter: A Nursing Treatment." American Journal
of Nursing 84 (1984): 991-992.

Hertzler, Joyce O. Laughter: A Socio-Scientific Analysis. New
York, NY: Exposition Press, 1970.

Holden, Robert. Laughter–The Best Medicine. London,
England: Thorsons, 1995.

Holland, Norman N. Laughing: A Psychology of Humor. Ithaca,
NY: Cornell Univ Press, 1982.

Holme, Bryan. A Present of Laughter. NY: Viking, 1982.

Hong, W. "Learning through Laughter: The Use of Cartoons in
Business Chinese." Journal of Language for International
Business 15.1 (2004): 100-116.

Humann, Ursula. "Der Witz als Waffe: Lachen und Humor in
der Jüdischen Tradition." Tribüne 126 (1993): 179-187.

Hudak, D., A. Dale, M. Hudak, and D. DeGood. "Effects of
Humorous Stimuli and Sense of Humor on Discomfort."
Psychological Reports 69.3 (1991): 779-786.

Hutcheson, Francis. Reflections on Laughter. New York, NY:
Garland, 1971.

Ishigami, S, A. Nakajima, M. Tanno, T. Matsuzaki, H. Suzuki,
and S. Yoshino. "Effects of Mirthful Laughter on Growth
Hormone, IGF-1 and Substance P in Patients with Rheumatoid
Arthritis." Clin. Exp. Rheumatol. 23.5 (2005): 651-657.

Jefferson, Gail. "An Exercise in the Transcription and Analysis
of Laughter." Handbook of Discourse Analysis, Volume 3:
Discourse and Dialogue. Ed. T. A. van Dijk. London, England:
Academic Press, 1985, 25-34.

Jefferson, Gail. "On the Organization of Laughter in Talk about
Troubles." Structures of Social Action: Studies in Conversational
Analysis. Eds. J. Atkinson and J. Heritage. Cambridge, England:
Cambridge University Press, 1984, 346-369.

Jefferson, Gail. "A Technique for Inviting Laughter and its
Subsequent Acceptance/Declination." Everyday Language:

Studies in Ethnomethodology. Ed. G. Psathas. New York, NY: Irvington, 1979, 79-96.

Jenkins, Ron. Subversive Laughter: the Liberating Power of Comedy. New York, NY: Free Press, 1994.

Johnson, Helen. "Counteracting Performaitivity in Schools: The Case for Laughter as a Qualitative and Redemptive Indicator." International Journal of Children's Spirituality 10.1 (2005): 81-96.

Joubert, Laurent. Treatise on Laughter. Trans. Gregory David de Rocher. Birmingham, AL: University of Alabama Press, 1980.

Juni, Samuel, and Bernard Katz. "Self-Effacing Wit as a Response to Oppression: Dynamics in Ethnic Humor." Journal of General Psychology Special Issue on Humor and Laughter Eds. Mahony, Diana L. and Louis G. Lippman.128.2 (2001): 117-119.

Kaplan, L. "Suspense, Para-Science and Laughter." Sub-Stance 71-71 (1993): 306-314.

Kasl, Charlotte Davis. Finding Joy. New York, NY: HarperCollins, 1994

Kataria, Madan. Laugh for No Reason. Mumbai, India Madhuri Press, 1999.

Kataria, Madan. Inner Spirit of Laughter, The. Bangalore, India, Dr Kataria School, 2012.

Karassev, Leonid V. Filosofia Smekha/Philosophy of Laughter. Moscow, Russia: R.G.G.U, 1996.

Kehl, D. G. "Varieties of Risible Experience: Grades of Laughter in Modern American Literature." HUMOR: International Journal of Humor Research 13.4 (2000): 279-395.

Kelly, K. "Laughter: A Hearty Har-Har." US News and World Report (March 21, 2005): 138-155.

Killeen, M. "Clinical Clowning: Humor in Hospice Care." American Journal of Hospice and Palliative Care 8.3 (1991).

Kimata, H. "Reduction of Allergic Responses in Atopic Infants by Mother's Laughter." European Journal of Clinical Investigation 34.9 (2004): 645-646.

Klein, Allen. The Healing Power of Humor. New York, NY: Tarcher/Putnam, 1989.

Kotani, K. "Socio-Psychological Activities Associated with Laughter in Older Japanese Females." Arch. Med. Res 37.1 (2006): 186-187.

Kraut, R. E., and R. E. Johnston. "Social and Emotional Messages of Smiling: An Ethological Approach." Journal of Personality Social Psychology. 37 (1979): 1539-1553.

Kreitler, H., and S. Kreitler. "Dependence of Laughter on Cognitive Strategies." Merrill-Palmer Quarterly 16 (April, 1970): 163-177.

Kuhn, C. C. "The Stages of Laughter." Journal of Nursing Jocularity 4.2 (1994): 34-35.

Kuipers, Giselinde. "Where Was King Kong When We Needed Him?: Public Discourse, Digital Disaster Jokes, and the Functions of Laughter after 9/11." Journal of American and Comparative Cultures 28.1 (2005): 70-84.

Kundera, Milan. The Book of Laughter and Forgetting. New York, NY: Penguin, 1980.

Kushner, B. "Laughter as Materiel: The Mobilization of Comedy in Japan's Fifteen-Year War." International History Review 26.2 (21004): 300-330.

LaFrance, M. "Felt Versus Feigned Funniness: Issues in Smiling and Laughing." Handbook of Humor Research I. Eds. P. G. McGhee, and J. H. Goldstein. New York, NY: Springer-Verlag, 1983, 1-12.

Labott, S., and R. Martin. "The Stress-Moderating Effects of Weeping and Humor." Journal of Human Stress 13.4 (1987).

Lahue, Kalton C. World of Laughter. Norman, OK: University of Oklahoma Press, 1966.

Lally, Steven. "Laugh Your Stress Away." Prevention. June, 1991: 50ff.

Lamb, Chris. "The Popularity of O. J. Simpson Jokes: The More We Know, the More We Laugh." Journal of Popular Culture 28.1 (1994): 223-232.

Lambert, R., and N. Lambert. "The Effects of Humor on Secretory Immunoglobulin A Levels in School-Aged Children." Pediatric Nursing 21.1 (1995): 16-19.

Lampert, Martin D., and Susan Ervin-Tripp. "Risky Laughter: Teasing and Self-Directed Joking among Male and Female Friends." Journal of Pragmatics, 38.1 (2006): 51-72.

Laura, Ronald S., and Bob Wolff. "Not Just for Laughs: Humor Can Relieve Stress and Prolong Life." Muscle and Fitness. December, 1992: 148ff.

Leclerc, Linda and Cosseron, Corinne Le Yoga du Rire (in French). Editions Trédaniel, Paris, France 2014

Leventhal, H., and W. Mace. "The Effect of Laughter on Evaluation of a Slapstick Movie." Journal of Personality 38 (1970): 16-30.

Levi, Primo. "Ritual and Laughter." Other People's Trades. New York, NY: Summit Books, 1989.

Lieber, D. B. "Laughter and Humor in Critical Care. Dimens Crit Care Nurs 5.3 (1986): 162-70.

Light, K. Humor as a Coping Strategy: Its Relationship to Role Strain in Women. M.A. Thesis. Tampa, FL: University of South Florida, 1997.

Lindvall, Terry. Surprised by Laughter. Nashville, TN: T. Nelson, 1996.

Lipman, Steve. Laughter in Hell: The Use of Humor during the Holocaust. Northvale, NJ: Jason Aronson, 1991.

Lippitt, John. "Nietzsche, Zarathustra and the Status of Laughter." British Journal of Aesthetics 32.1 (1992).

Littleton, J. "Learning to Laugh, and Laughing to Learn." Montessori Life 10 (1998): 42-44.

Long, Patricia. "Laugh and Be Well?" Psychology Today 21.10 (1987): 28-29.

Loomans, D., and K. J. Kolberg. The Laughing Classroom: Everyone's Guide to Teaching with Humor and Play. Tiburon, CA: H. J. Kramer, 1993.

Lowe, G., and S. B. Taylor. "Relationship between Laughter and Weekly Alcohol Consumption." Psychological Reports 72.3 (1993): 1210

Ludovici, Anthony M. The Secret of Laughter. London, England: Constable Press, 1932.

Lundell, Torborg. "An Experiential Exploration of Why Men and Women Laugh." HUMOR: International Journal of Humor Research 6.3 (1993): 299-318.

McAdams, D. P., R. J. Jackson, and C. Kirshmit. "Looking, Laughing, and Smiling in Dyads as a Function of Intimacy Motivations and Reciprocity." Journal of Personality. 52.3 (1984): 261-273.

McGhee, Paul E. The Laughter Remedy: Health, Healing, and the Amuse System. Randolph, New Jersey: Paul McGhee 1991.

MacDonald, C.M. "A chuckle a day keeps the doctor away: therapeutic humor and laughter." Journal of Psychosocial Nursing and Mental Health services, 42(3), 18-25. 2004

MacHovec, F. "Humor in Therapy." Psychotherapy in Private Practice 9.1 (1991): 25-33.

McMahon, C., A. Mahmud, and J. Freely. "Taking Blood Pressure–No Laughing Matter!" Blood Pressur Monitor 10.2 (2005): 109-110.

Machline, Vera Cecelia. "The Legend Behind the Epithet 'Sardonic Laugh,' 2000 Ans de Rire: Permanence et Modernite ed. Mongi Medina. Besançons, France: Presses Universitaires France-Comtoises, 2002, 77-86.

Mager, M., and P. A. Cabe. "Is Propensity to Laugh Equivalent to Sense of Humor?" Psychological Reports 66.3 (1990): 737-738.

Mahony, Diana L., and M. D. Corson. "Light-Mindedness versus Lightheartedness: Conflicting Conceptions of Laughter among Latter-Day Saints." BYU Studies 42.2 (2003): 115-129.

Mahony, Diana L., W. Jeffrey Burroughs, and Arron C. Hieatt. "The Effects of Laughter on Discomfort Thresholds: Does Expectation Become Reality?" Journal of General Psychology "Special Issue on Humor and Laughter" Eds. Mahony, Diana L. and Louis G. Lippman.128.2 (2001): 217-226.

Mahony, Diana L. and Louis G. Lippman, eds. "Introduction to the Special Issue on 'Humor and Laughter.'" Journal of General Psychology 128.2 (2001): 117-119.

Mallett, Jane. "Humour and Laughter Therapy." The Nurses' Handbook of Complementary Therapies. London, England: Churchill-Livingston, 1995, 109-117.

Mallett, Jane. "The Use of Humour and Laughter in Patient Care." British Journal of Nursing. 2 (1993): 172-175.

Mandel, Siegfried. "The Laughter of Nordic and Celtic Irish Tricksters." Fabula 23.1-2 (1982): 35-47.

Marmysz, John. Laughing at Nothing: Humor as a Response to Nihilism. Albany, NY: SUNY Press, 2003.

Martin, G. Neil, and Colin D. Gray. "The Effects of Audience Laughter on Men's and Women's Responses to Humor." Journal of Social Psychology 136.2 (1996): 221-231.

Martin, Rod A. "Humor, Laughter, and Physical Health: Methodological Issues and Research Findings." Psychological Bulletin 127.4 (2001): 504-519.

Martin, Rod, N. Kuiper, J. Olinger, and K. Dance. "Humor, Coping with Stress, Self Concept, and Psychological Well-being." HUMOR: International Journal of Humor Research 6.1 (1993): 89-104.

Martin, R.A. "Is laughter the best medicine?" Current Directions in Psychological science, 11, 216-220, 2002.

Martin, Rod A. The Psychology of Humor: An Integrative Approach Burlington, MA: Elsevier Academic Press, 2007.

Martin, Rod, and Herbert Lefcourt. "Sense of Humor as a Moderator of the Relation between Stressors and Mood." Journal of Personality and Social Psychology 45 (1983): 1313-1324.

Meyer, M., S. Zysset, D. Y. von Cramon, and K. Alter. "Distinct fMRI Responses to Laughter, Speech, and Sounds along the Human Peri-Sylvian Cortex." Cognitive Brain Research 24.2 (2005): 291-306.

Mills, Letha. "Laughter is the Best Medicine." Active Years 14 (2002): 74-77.

Milner, George B. "Homo Ridens: Towards a Semiotic Theory of Humor and Laughter." Semiotica 5 (1972): 1-30.

Miyamoto, Lance. "Why Laughing is Good for You." Science Digest. June, 1981, 27.

Monro, D. H. Argument of Laughter. Notre Dame, IN: University of Notre Dame Press, 1963.

Morreall, John. "Humor and Laughter." Encyclopedia of U.S. Popular Culture. Forthcoming.

Morreall, John. "Laughter." Encyclopaedia Britannica, Japanese Edition. Forthcoming.

Morreall, John. "Laughter, Suddenness, and Pleasure." Dialogue: Canadian Philosophical Review 23 (1984): 689-694.

Morreall, John. "A New Theory of Laughter." The Philosophy of Laughter and Humor. Ed. John Morreall. Albany, NY: SUNY Press, 1987, 128-38.

Morreall, John. Taking Laughter Seriously. Albany, NY: SUNY Press, 1983.

Mowrer, Donald E. "A Case Study of Perceptual and Acoustic Features of an Infant's First Laugh Utterances." HUMOR: International Journal of Humor Research 7.2 (1994): 139-156.

Mueller, Rolph, and Guenter Braus. "Laughter," Special Issue of High Quality: Magazine of Design and Printing 22.1 (1992). Heidelberg, Germany: Rosi Pluschke-Moser; NOTE: There is also a German version.

Mulkay, Michael, Colin Clark, and Trevor Pinch. "Laughter and the Profit Motive: The Use of Humor in a Photographic Shop." HUMOR: International Journal of Humor Research. 6.2 (1993): 163-194.

Mulkay, Michael, and Gerard Howe. "Laughter for Sale." The Sociological Review 42.3 (1994): 481-500.

Nasir, U. M., S. Iwanaga, Ahmn Nabi, O. Urayama, K. Hayashi, T. Hayashi, K. Kawai, A. Sultana, K. Murakami, and F. Suzuki. "Laughter Therapy Modulates the Parameters of Renin-

Angiotensin System in Patients with Type 2 Diabetes." International Journal of Molecular Medicine 16.6 (2005): 1077-1082.

Nerhardt, G. "Humor and Inclination to Laugh: Emotional Reactions to Stimuli of Different Divergence from a Range of Expectancy." Scandinavian Journal of Psychology 11 (1970): 185-95.

Neuendorf, Kimberley, and Tom Fennell. "A Social Facilitation View of the Generation of Humor and Mirth Reactions: Effects of a Laugh Track." Central States Speech Journal 39.1 (1988): 37-48.

Nichols, Stephen G. "Laughter as Gesture: Hilarity and the Anti-Sublime." Neohelicon 32.2 (2005): 375-389.

Niebylski, Dianna C. Humoring Resistance: Laughter and the Excessive Body in Contemporary Women's Fiction, Albany, NY: State University of New York Press, 2004.

Niles, R. "Wigs, Laughter, and Subversion: Charles Busch and Strategies of Drag Performance." Journal of Homosexuality 46.3-4 (2004): 35-54.

Nilsen, Alleen Pace, and Don L. F. Nilsen. "Laughter and Smiles." Encyclopedia of 20th Century American Humor. Westport, CT: Greenwood Press, 2000, 184-186.

Nilsen, Don L. F. "Laughter and Smiling." Humor Scholarship: A Research Bibliography. Westport, CT: Greenwood, 1993, 1-5.

Nwokah, Eva E. "Giggle Time in the Infant/Toddler Classroom: Learning and Connecting Through Shared Humor and Laughter." Focus on Infants and Toddlers 16.2 (2003): 1-8.

Nwokah, Evangeline, and Alan Fogel. "Laughter in Mother-Infant Emotional Communication." HUMOR: International Journal of Humor Research. 6.2 (1993): 137-162.

O'Donnell-Trujillo, Nick, and Katherine Adams. "Heheh in Conversation: Some Coordinating Accomplishments of Laughter." The Western Journal of Speech Communications 47 (Spring 1983): 175-191.

Okun, M. S., D. Bowers, U. Springer, N. A. Shapira, D. Malone, A. R. Rezai, B. Nuttin, K. M. Heilman, R. J. Morecraft, S. A. Rasmussen, B. D. Greenberg, K. D. Foote, and W. K. Goodman." Neurocase 10.4 (2004): 271-279.

Osaka, N., and M. Osaka. "Striatal Reward Areas Activated by Implicit Laughter Induced by Mimic Words in Humans: A Functional Magnetic Resonance Imaging Study." Neuroreport 16.15 (2005): 1621-1624.

Osho. Joy: The Happiness that Comes from Within. New York, NY: St. Martin's Griffin, 2004.

Osho. Life, Love, Laughter. Nepal: Osho Tapoban Pubications, Overeem, Sebastian, Walter Taal, E. Öcal Gezici, Gert Jan Lammers, and J. Gert van Dijk. "Is Motor Inhibition during Laughter due to Emotional or Respiratory Influences?" Pscychophysiology 41.2 (2004): 254ff.

Owren, M. J., and J-A Bachorowski. "Reconsidering the Evolution of Nonlinguistic Communication: The Case of Laughter." Journal of Nonverbal Behavior 27.3 (2003): 183-200.

Padus, Emrika. The Complete Guide to Your Emotions and Your Health. Emmaus, Pennsylvania: Rodale Press, 1986.

Parse, R. R. "Laughing and Health–A Study Using Parse Research Method." Nursing Science Quarterly 123.2 (1994): 129-145.

Paskind, J. "Effects of Laughter on Muscle Tone." Archives of Neurology and Psychiatry 28 (1932): 623-628.

Pasquali, Elaine Anne. "Learning to Laugh: Humor as Therapy." Journal of Psychosocial Nursing 28.3 (March, 1990): 31-35.

Paul, William. Laughing Screaming: Modern Hollywood Horror and Comedy. New York, NY: Columbia University Press, 1994.

Pepper, Melissa. "In Outer Space No One Can Hear Your Laughter." Australian Journal of Comedy 2 (1995): 101-114.

Petithory, Frédérique. Le yoga du rire en 99 definitions (in French). Nice, France: Editions Bénévent, 2006.

Peter, Laurence, and Bill Dana. The Laughter Prescription. New York, NY: Ballentine, 1982.

Pfeifer, Karl. "Laughter and Pleasure." HUMOR: International Journal of Humor Research 7 (1994): 157-172.

Pfeifer, Karl. "Laughter, Freshness and Titillation." Inquiry 40 (1997): 307-322.

Pfeifer, Karl. "From Locus Neoclassicus to Locus Rattus: Notes on Laughter, Comprehensiveness, and Titillation. " Res Cogitans 3 (2006) 29-46.

Pfeifer, Karl. "More on Morreall on Laughter." Dialogue 26 (1987): 161-166.

Piddington, Ralph. The Psychology of Laughter. New York, NY: Gamut Press, 1963.

Pink, Daniel. A Whole New Mind: Why Right-Brainers will Rule the Future. New York, NY: Penguin, 2005.

Plessner, Helmuth. Laughing and Crying. Evanston, IL: Northwestern University Press, 1970.

Podlichak, Walter. "Fun, Funny, Fun–Of Humor and Laughter." Humor: International Journal of Humor Research. 5.4 (1992): 375-396.

Polio, Howard R., Rodney Mers, and William Lucchesi. "Humor, Laughter, and Smiling: Some Preliminary Observations of Funny Behaviors." The Psychology of Humor. Eds. Jeffrey Goldstein and Paul McGhee. NY: Academic Press, 1972,2 211-42.

Porteous, Janice. "Humor as a Process of Defense: The Evolution of Laughing." Humor: International Journal of Humor Research 1.1 (1988): 63-80.

Powell, B. S. "Laughter and Healing: The Use of Humor in Hospitals Treating Children." J Assoc Care Child Hosp 3.2 (1974): 10-16.

Poyatos, F. "Many Voices of Laughter–A New Audible-Visual Paralinguistic Approach." Semiotica 93.1-2 (1993): 61-81.

Prakash, Vishwa. Who Stole my Soul? Austin, TX: Synergy Books, 2009.

Prerost, F. "Presentation of Humor and Facilitation of a Relaxation Response among Internal and External Scores on Rotter's Scale." Psychological Reports 72 (1993): 1248-1250.

Prerost, F. "Use of Humor and Guided Imagery in Therapy to Alleviate Stress." Journal of Mental Health Counseling 10.1 (1988): 16-22.

Propp, Vladimir. "Ritual Laughter in Folklore." Theory and History of Folklore. Minneapolis, MN: University of Minnesota, 1984.

Provine, Robert R. "Contagious Laughter: Laughter is a Sufficient Stimulus for Laughs and Smiles." Bulletin of the Psychonomic Society 30.1 (1992): 1-4.

Provine, Robert R. "Contagious Yawning and Laughter." Social Learning in Animals: The Roots of Culture. Eds. C. M. Heyes, and B. G. Galef. New York, NY: Academic Press, 1996.

Provine, Robert R. "The Laughing Species." Natural History December, 2000, 72-77.

Provine, Robert R. "Laughing, Tickling, and the Evolution of Speech and Self." Current Directions in Psychological Science 13.6 (2004): 215-218.

Provine, Robert R. "Laughter." American Scientist 84.1 (1996).

Provine, Robert R. "Laughter: A Novel Tool for Understanding Vocal Production, Perceptions, and Social Behavior." American Scientist 84.1 (1996): 38-40

Provine, Robert R. Laughter: A Scientific Investigation. New York, NY: Harmondsworth/Penguin, 2001.

Provine, Robert R. "Laughter Punctuates Speech: Linguistic, Social and Gender Contexts of Laughter." Ethology 95.4 (1993): 291-298.

Provine, Robert R., and Kenneth R. Fischer. "Laughing, Smiling, and Talking: Relation to Sleeping and Social Context in Humans." Ethology 83 (1989): 295-305.

Provine, Robert R., and Yvonne L. Young. "Laughter: A Stereotyped Human Vocalization." Ethology 89 (1991): 115-124.

Ransohoff, R. "Some Observations on Humor and Laughter in Young Adolescent Girls." Journal of Youth and Adolescence 4 (1975): 155-170.

Raskin, Victor. "Better to Laugh: Linking Humor, Creativity, and Intelligence." The World and I (June, 1992): 658-660.

Repplier, Agnes. In Pursuit of Laughter. Boston, MA: Houghton Mifflin, 1936.

Rothbart, Mary K. "Incongruity, Problem-Solving and Laughter." Humor and Laughter: Theory, Research, and Applications. Eds. Antony J. Chapman, and Hugh C. Foot. New Brunswick, NJ: Transaction, 1996, 37-54.

Rothbart, Mary K. "Laughter in Young Children." Psycholigical Bulletin 80.3 (1973): 247-256.

Ruch, Willibald. "Commentary." Charles Darwins' Expression of Emotions in Man and Animals (3rd Edition). Ed. Paul Ekman. New York, NY: Oxford University Press, 1998.

Ruch, Willibald. "Extraversion, Alcohol, and Enjoyment." What the Face Reveals: Basic and Applied Studies of Spontaneous Expression Using the Facial Action Coding System. Eds. Paul Ekman, and E. L. Rosenberg. Oxford, England: Oxford University Press, 1997, 112-130.

Ruch, Willibald. "The FACS in Humor Research." What the Face Reveals: Basic and Applied Studies of Spontaneous Expression Using the Facial Action Coding System. Eds. Paul Ekman, and E. L. Rosenberg. Oxford, England: Oxford University Press, 1997, 109-111.

Ruch, Willibald. "Laughter and Temperament." What the Face Reveals: Basic and Applied Studies of Spontaneous Expression

149

Using the Facial Action Coding System. Eds. P. Ekman, and E. L. Rosenberg. Oxford, England: Oxford University Press, 1997.

Ruch, Willibald, and Lambert Deckers. "Do Extroverts Like to Laugh? An Analysis of the Situational Humor Response Questionnaire." European Journal of Personality 7.4 (1993).

Ruch, Willibald, and P. Ekman. "The Expressive Pattern of Laughter." Emotion, Qualia, and Consciousness. Tokyo, Japan: Word Scientific Publisher, 2001.

Russell, Roy E. Life, Mind and Laughter: A Theory of Laughter. Chicago, IL: Adams Press, 1987.

Russell, Roy E. "Understanding Laughter in Terms of Basic Perceptual and Response Patterns." HUMOR: International Journal of Humor Research 9.1 (1996): 39-56.

Rutter, Jason. Stand-Up as Interaction: Performance and Audience in Comedy Venues. Unpublished Ph.D. Dissertation. Salford, England: University of Salford, 1997.

Ruxton, J., and M. Hesler. "Humor: Assessment and Interventions." Clinical Gerontologist 7.1 (1987): 13-21.

Salamone, Frank A. "Laughin' Louie: An Analysis of Louis Armstrong's Record and its Relationship to African-American Musical Humor." HUMOR: International Journal of Humor Research 15.1 (2002): 47-64.

Sanders, Barry. Laughter as Subversive History. Boston, MA: Beacon Press, 1995.

Sanders, T. "Controllable Laughter: Managing Sex Work through Humour." Sociology 38.2 (2004): 273-291.

Satow, R. "Three Perspectives on Humor and Laughing–Classical, Object, Relations and Self Psychology." Group 15.4 (1991): 242-245.

Schaeffer, Neil. The Art of Laughter. New York: Columbia Univ Press, 1981.

Scherberger, L. "The Janus-Faced Shaman: The Role of Laughter in Sickness and Healing among the Makushi." Anthropology and Humanism 30.1 (2005): 55-69.

Schickel, Richard. The Shape of Laughter. Boston, MA: New York Graphics Society, 1974.

Schopenhauer, Arthur. "On the Theory of the Ludicrous." The World as will and Idea. Trans. R. B. Haldane and John Kemp. London, England: Routledge and Kegan Paul, 1907.

Schulman, N. M. "Laughing across the Color Barrier: In Living Color–Satirizing the Stereotypes–Racial Generalization as a Basis for Comedy." Journal of Popular Film and Television 20.1 (1992).

Scruton, Roger. "Laughter." The Philosophy of Laughter and Humor. Ed. John Morreall. Albany, NY: SUNY, 1987, 156-171.

Scruton, Roger. "Laughter." Proceedings of the Aristotelian Society 56 (1982).

Shapiro, Rebecca. R. D. V. Glasgow: Madness, Masks, and Laughter. Teaneck, NJ: Farleigh Dickinson University Press, 1995.

Sheldon, S. T. "Tickle." Journal of the American Academy of Dermatology. 50 (2004): 93-97.

Shoji, Osamu. "Study of Dr. Sutorius' Theory Concerning Laughter." The Journal of Ryutsu Keizai University 34.3 (2000).

Simon, John Charles. Why We Laugh: a new understanding. Carmel, IN: Starbook Publishing 2008.

Simon, Jolene. "Humor and the Older Adult: Implications for Nursing." Journal of Advanced Nursing Practice 13 (1988).

Simon, Jolene. "Humor Techniques for Oncology Nurses." Oncology Nursing Forum 16.5 (19789): 667-670.

Smith, J. "The Frenzy of the Audible: Pleasure, Authenticity, and Recorded Laughter." Television and New Media 6.1 (2005).

Smith, Ken. "Laughing at the Way We See: The Role of Visual Organizing Principles in Cartoon Humor." HUMOR: International Journal of Humor Research 9.1 (1996): 19-38.

Sobel, David S. and Ornstein, Robert. The Healthy Mind Healthy Body Handbook. New York, NY: Time Life Medical, 1996.

Solomon, Robert. "Are the Three Stooges Funny? Soitainly! (or When is it OK to Laugh?)." Ethics and Values in the Information Age. Eds. Joel Rudinow and Anthony Graybosch. New York, NY: Wadsworth, 2002.

Spencer, Herbert. "The Physiology of Laughter." MaclMillan's Magazine 1 (1860).

Spitz, R. "The Smiling Response: A Contribution to the Ontogenesis of Social Relations." General Psychology Monograph 34 (1946): 57-125.

Strack, F., L. Martin, and S. Strepper. "Inhibiting and Facilitating Conditions of the Human Smile: A Nonobtrusive Test of the Facial-Feedback Hypothesis." Journal of Personality and Social Psychology 54 (1988): 768-777.

Stearns, F. R. Laughing: Physiology, Pathology, Psychology, Pathopsychology and Development. Springfield, IL: Charles C. Thomas, 1972.

151

Stebbins, Robert A. The Laugh-Makers: Stand-Up Comedy as Art, Business, and Life-Style. Montreal: McGill-Queen's University Press, 1990.

Sterling, Philip. Laughing on the Outside. NY: Grosset and Dunlap, 1965.

Stone, Judith. "Laugh and Your Whole Cardiovascular System Laughs with You–Not to Mention Your Stress Hormones." In Health. 5 (January, 1992): 52-55.

Strean, Billy. The HoHo Dojo. Edmonton, AB Canada

Stroufe, L. A., and E. Waters. "The Ontogenesis of Smiling and Laughter: A Perspective on the Organization of Development in Infancy." Psychological Review 83.3 (1976): 173-189.

Stroufe, L. A., and J. P. Wunsch. "The Development of Laughter in the First Year of Life." Child Development 43 (1972).

Sully, J. An Essay on Laughter. New York, NY: Longmans/Green, 1902.

Sumitsuji, N., and Y. Takemura. "Electromyography Counting of the Numbers of Times of the Laughing Act in Man." Electromyography 1 (1971): 55-60.

Svebak, Sven. "Three Attitude Dimensions of Sense of Humor as Predictors of Laughter." Scandinavian Journal of Psychology 15 (1974): 185-190.

Svebak, Sven, and Michael J. Apter. "Laughter: An Empirical Test of Some Reversal Theory Hypotheses." Scandinavian Journal of Psychology 28 (1987): 189-198.

Swabey, Mary Collins. "Comic Laughter: A Philosophical Essay." New Haven, CT: Yale University Press, 1961.

Tamblyn, Doni. Laugh and Learn: 95 Ways to Use Humor for More Effective Teaching and Training. New York, NY: AMACON (American Management Association), 2003.

Tarantili, V. V. D. J. Halazonetis, and M. N. Spyropoulos. "The Spontaneous Smile in Dynamic Motion." American Journal of Dentofacial Orthop 128.1 (2005): 8-15.

Taylor, Paul. "Laughter and Joking–The Structural Axis." It's a Funny Thing, Humour. Eds. Antony Chapman and Hugh Foot. NY: Pergamon, 1977, 385-90.

Thorson, James A. "Is Propensity to Laugh Equivalent to Sense of Humor?" Psychological Reports 66.3 (1990): 737-738.

Toren, C. "Laughter and Truth in Fiji: What We May Learn from a Joke." Oceania 75.3 (2005): 268-283.

Trice, A., and J. Price. "Joking under the Drill: A Validity Study of the Coping Humor Scale." Journal of Social Behavior and Personality 1.2 (1986): 265-266.

Trieber, Roz. Live Life Laughing: An Innovative and Imaginative Approach to Living a Healthier, Happier, and More Prosperous Life. Owings Mills, MD: Trieber Associates, 2000.

Vaid, Jyotsna. "Do Those Who Laugh Last? The Evolution of Humor." Evolution of the Psyche. Eds. D. Rosen, and M. Luebbert. Westport, CT: Greenwood, 1999.

Vaid, Jyotsna. "Laughter and Humor." Encyclopedia of the Human Brain. Ed. V. S. Ramachandran. Academic Press, 2000.

Vaid, Jyotsna. "Laughter and Humor." Oxford Companion to the Body Eds. C. Blakemore and S. Jennett. Oxford, England: Oxford University Press, 2001, 426-427.

Vaid, Jyotsna, and J. B. Kobler. "Laughing Matters: Toward a Structural and Neural Account." Brain and Cognition 42 (2000).

Van Hoof, J. A. R. A. M. "A Comparative Approach to the Phylogeny of Laughter and Smiling." Non-Verbal Communication. Ed. R. A. Hinds. Cambridge, England: University Press.

Vettin, Julia, and Dietmar Todt. "Laughter in Conversation: Features of Occurence and Acoustic Structure." Journal of Nonverbal Behavior. 28.2 (2004): 93-115

Viktoroff, David. Introduction à la Psycho-Sociologie du Rire. Paris, France: Presses Universitaires de France, 1953.

Wallace, Earle Stegner. Remembering Laughter. Boston, MA: Little Brown, 1937.

Weeks, Mark C. "Laughter, Desire, and Time." HUMOR: International Journal of Humor Research. 15.4 (2002): 383-400.

Weisfeld, G. E. "Adaptive Value of Humor and Laughter." Ethology and Sociobiology 14.2 (1993): 141-169.

Weiskrantz, L. J., Elliott, and C. Darlington. "Preliminary Observations on Tickling Oneself." Nature 230 (1970): 598-599.

Westbrook, Kathy Grant. "Laugh It Up: Carolina Ha Ha Prescribes a Healthy Dose of Humor to Combat Pain and Stress and to Help Folks Feel More Positive." Our State: Down Home in North Carolilna, (January, 2005): 62-64.

Whistler, Laurence. Laughter and the Urn: The Life of Rex Whistler. NY: Wiedenfeld and Nicolson, 1985.

White, Sabina, and Andrew Winzelberg. "Laughter and Stress." Humor: International Journal of Humor Research. 5.4 (1992).

White, Sabina, and P. Camarena. "Laughter as a Stress Reducer in Small Groups." HUMOR: International Journal of Humor Research 2.1 (1989): 73-79.

Williams, H. "Humor and Healing: Therapeutic Effects in Geriatrics." Gerontion 1.3 (1986): 14-17.

Willman, J. M. "An Analysis of Humor and Laughter." American Journal of Psychology 53 (1940).

Wise, B. "Comparison of Immune Response to Mirth and to Distress in Women at Risk for Recurrent Breast Cancer." Dissertation Abstracts International 49.7 (1989): 2918.

Wolosin, R. J. "Cognitive Similarity and Group Laughter." Journal of Personality and Social Psychology 32 (1975): 505-509.

Wooten, Patty. Compassionate Laughter: Jest for Your Health. New York, NY: Commune-a-Key, 1996.

Ziegler, J. "Immune System May Benefit from the Ability to Laugh." Journal of the National Cancer Institute 87.5 (1995).

Zijderveld, Anton C. "The Sociology of Humour and Laughter." Current Sociology 31.3 (1983): 1-103.

Zijderveld, Anton C. "Trend Report on the Sociology of Humor and Laughter." Current Sociology 31.3 (1983): 1-59.

....

Answers to the Laughter Yoga Exam (p. 97-100)

1 = b; in collaboration with his lovely wife, Madhuri. **2 = d**. **3 = c. 4 = e. 5 = b. 6 = a. 7 = d**; give yourself 0.1 point if you guessed 'Madman' – a nickname Dr. Kataria may have been given when he first proposed laughing for no reason ("Are you crazy, Doc?"). **8 = f**; your author was a spokesperson for Laughter Yoga in all of the media listed. **9 = e. 10 = d**; extra credit if you know which Neil Simon play has the "Words with Letter K are what's funny" routine, and/or if you know the proper de-euphemization of "Particularly Nasty Weather". **11 = e**; regarding letter d, we never want to say negative comments, like "No", "Stop", or "Wrong". These may reactivate traumatic childhood experiences when laughter was suppressed or even punished. Instead, we want to lead the participant to a *positive* experience of what is next, such as: the pleasurable chant/clap of "Ho, ho, ha-ha-ha", words of encouragement, or the introduction to the next fun Laughter Exercise.

Resources

(USA and the World)

BOOKS (the essentials)

Gesundheit! (Adams)

- *The Laughter Yoga Book*
- *The Great Big Anthology of Laughter Exercises*

Laughter Revolutionaries (Briar)

(For Gibberish:) *Froigen deebled Craggle-zorp! - The All-Gibberish Photo- and Story-book* (Briar)

Anatomy of an Illness (as Perceived by the Patient); Head First (Cousins)

- *Laugh For No Reason* (Kataria)

The Psychology of Humor (Martin)

VIDEOS

Laughter Bank volumes 1, 2, 3 (and many more) (Kataria)

The Laughter Club in Real Time; Gibberish Sets You Free! (Briar)

CONTACTS

Headquarters (Laughter Yoga University and Laughter Yoga International Foundation) :
www.LaughterYoga.org
Email: help@laughteryoga.org

The Laughter Yoga Institute : www.LYInstitute.org
790 Manzanita Drive, Laguna Beach, CA 92651-1962
USA
Phone/fax: (949) 376-1939   Mobilephone: (949) 315-5801   Email: JoyfulB@cox.net

Laugh4Health YahooGroup :
http://health.groups.yahoo.com/group/Laugh4Health/

ONLINE VIDEOS

All available on YouTube (free):
Five Minute Warm-Up - Laughter Club
Gibberish 101 - How to Speak Gibberish
Gibberish Instructional Videos (many)
The Ho Ho Ha Ha Laughter Club March
The Laughalong March
Laughter as Aerobic Exercise (with Norma Schechtman)
Laughter Club: Beach Laughing, How We Do It in Laguna

The Laughter Club Song ("Come to the Laughter Club")
Laughter Kirtan
Laughter Exercise Videos (many). See YouTube channels "Joyful Gent" and "Jeffrey Briar"

QUOTES ON LAUGHTER : http://lyinstitute.org/quotes-on-laughter/

BUSINESS Cards and Literature, Personalized Products

To self-publish Books, audio CDs, DVDs (affiliated with Amazon.com): www.createspace.com

Many promotional items/business cards free, pay only shipping: www.vistaprint.com

Low cost printing, more choices:
www.overnightprints.com

T-shirts, caps (embroidery, printing):
www.queensboro.com

Custom shirts, stickers, artwork:
www.happylifeproductions.com

Laughter Exercise Photo Flash Cards (files, you print):
http://lyinstitute.org/store/

Liability Insurance

We register as "Yoga Teachers" with a specialization in
Laughter Yoga; currently under $200 per year for One
Million Dollars' Coverage.

2. Sports & Fitness Insurance   www.sportsfitness.com
PO Box 1967   Madison, MS 39130-1967   800-844-0536

3. Fitness and Wellness Insurance Agency
   www.phly.com/products/FWI_Home.aspx
380 Stevens Avenue, Suite 206   Solana Beach, CA 92075
   800-395-8075

Professional Associations

Most have conferences.

AATH (Association for Applied Therapeutic Humor)
   www.aath.org

ISHS (International Society for Humor Studies):
   www.hnu.edu/ishs

Laughter Yoga Prozone: Write to
   laugh@laughteryoga.org

Laughter Yoga Conferences: See International
   Headquarters' website www.laughteryoga.org

PROZONE a service from Laughter Yoga University (International Headquarters)

exclusively for certified Laughter Yoga Leaders and Teachers. Initial membership with limited benefits is free to graduates of Leader and Teacher training. For full benefits there is a low annual fee.

Express your professional commitment to Laughter Yoga. You receive special e-mail newsletters from Dr. Kataria, advance notice of upcoming programs and products from L.Y. International, discount offers on L.Y. International products, and registration in a members-only facebook page frequented by Dr. Kataria and all the top Laughter Yoga professionals in the world.

➤ For completion of the 2-day Certified Laughter Yoga **Leader** Training: You receive a 1-year partial membership, with limited benefits, at no charge. Paying the annual fee gives you *free* an added **six months** of PROZONE membership with full benefits. In other words: When you purchase one year's membership at the current fee, you receive an additional six months at no additional charge. Full benefits include the opportunity for you to announce your fee-charging laughter-related programs, retreats, trainings and workshops on the international website.

➤ With completion of the 5-day (minimum) Certified Laughter Yoga **Teacher** Training: You receive a 1-year partial membership, with limited benefits, at no charge. Paying the annual fee gives you *free* an added year - **twelve months** - of PROZONE membership with full benefits. In other words: When you purchase one year's membership at the current fee, you receive a second year at no additional charge.

(All terms above are subject to change without notice from international headquarters in India.)

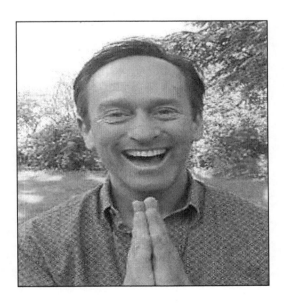

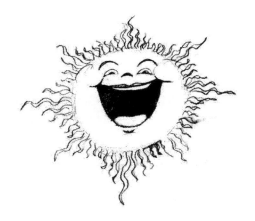

Early draft of "Lenny the Laughing Sun"

mascot for Laguna Laughter Club

by Lynn Kubasek

AFTERWORD — A Request

I sincerely hope you enjoyed the *Laughter Mastery* collection. Now I feel the need to express my concern about recent developments in the Laughter Yoga field.

We've seen efforts to add practices from disciplines such as Positive Psychology, Games Theory, Hypnotherapy, Brain Fitness, Improvisational and Rehearsed Theater, Singing and other Respiratory Therapies, Modern/Intuitive Dance, etc. Activities from these fields may be valuable and therapeutic, yet they may not be appropriate for a session which is dedicated to unconditional hearty laughing.

Some laughter exercise leaders become so enamored of these techniques that they offer them while neglecting the fundamental purpose of a Laughter Yoga session, which is: for people to laugh. However, **in order to get the health benefits of laughter, people need to actually *laugh*.** (We need only 10-15 minutes of laughter time to transform our chemistry and achieve the major health benefits.)

Some of the practices which are currently widespread include:

> singing songs, playing games, sharing jokes, telling stories, talking in gibberish, Improv and other theater games, mime sketches, psychological cathartic exercises, dancing (both choreographed and free-form), contests and competitions.

While these activities may be enjoyable and even therapeutic, they do not provide the benefits specific to laughing. Sessions without prolonged laughter do not deliver on the promises made in the "Three Reasons to Do Laughter Yoga" (p.18): #1, *Duration*, laughing for a prolonged period of time (**"We need to laugh continuously for at least 10 to 15 minutes" -- Dr. Kataria**); and #3, *Dependability* (**"We are not leaving laughter to chance, but doing it out of commitment" -- Dr. Kataria**). During the aforementioned practices, there may be little or no laughter at all for extended periods of time. Acting out a theater game, pretending to scrape the emotion of "Frustration" off our shoulders, performing a folkdance – these generally do not occur to the sound of prolonged abundant laughter.

Let me share from my personal experience. In my youth, my classmates shamed and teased me about my poor singing abilities, as well as my lack of proficiency in sports/games. In my adult years, I attended many psychology and theater workshops. When techniques from these outside disciplines are brought into a laughter session, a whole new set of filters and judgments arise. If a laughter session leader announces we are going to be singing songs, playing a competitive game, or dredging up negative emotional baggage from our past, I cringe. My happiness level plummets. I want to get out.

And a Laughter Yoga session without laughter is a sorrowful and disappointing affair.

These outside practices can be great to offer as a warm-up *before* the laughter session, or as an activity to enjoy *after* the laughing time; or on a separate date as part of a workshop or special event. If a person like me really doesn't want to participate, they can leave - while the others sing, learn the choreography, are instructed in the rules of the game, etc.

A few of these practices could be successfully adapted to facilitate plentiful voluntary laughter. Examples: a game like Follow the Leader, where the leader does a Laughter Exercise and the others follow them (thus, the participants are laughing – p. 28); or Gibberish Punchlines (p. 34-35) where a few moments of spoken gibberish result in a prolonged period of laughter. If there is abundant laughing involved, such activities would be welcome during a laughter segment. But if practices do not include laughter, or are dependent on strategizing or memorizing, let such be offered at a time outside the laughter segment.

Laughter Yoga friends in Hungary handled this in a responsible way.

They announced a weekly 2-hour session. The first 50 minutes consisted of Laughter Yoga (offered free of charge), with introduction, body warm-up, laughter exercises, Laughter Meditation, and Guided Relaxation (Yoga Nidra). Then there was a 15-minute break, with coffee, tea and socializing.

After the break, a Dance Class was offered. The

style of dance changed each week. One week there were lessons in Swing Dancing; another week, Hungarian Folk Dance, etc. The second session required a fee of $10 per person, most of which went to the dance instructor.

A few people attended only the Laughter Yoga portion. They left during the break. A few others arrived after the break and attended only the Dance Class. In this way, the laughter session was whole and complete, and the dance class was clearly outside – specifically, *after* - the laughter session.

Kathryn Burns tells us about attending a regular gathering in Bali where they do Laughter Yoga for a full hour, then they take a refreshment break, and then there is dancing for a second hour. The dance segment has plenty of laughter - sometimes spontaneous, sometimes guided. But if a person didn't want to dance (or was physically unable to), they were able to enjoy the full benefits of a complete laughter session by attending the first hour of the evening. (Kathy's full story can be found in the book *Laughter Revolutionaries*.)

My humble request is that we be certain to always fill our laughter sessions *with laughing*. (Remember, this need only be 10 to 15 minutes of hilarity to receive laughter's benefits.) For other "outside" practices, please: offer them outside the laughter segment.

With Love and Laughter, Sincerely,

Jeffrey Briar   November 14, 2017

Rashid's Surprise Package

A Bonus Adventure-Story from Jeffrey Briar

(Written as fiction; possibly true.)

The Divided "City of Peace"

In Jerusalem in early summer, the sun stubbornly refuses to set before 7:30pm. Rashid was wishing he could change that. He wanted the blanket of darkness to hide his actions from those around him: on his side of the fence, so no one would try to dissuade him from his task; and on the other side especially, where he would likely be discouraged with greater malice. Most of the border guards carried TAVOR assault rifles.

He walked purposefully at first. But as he approached the street with the dividing wall at its end he began to hunker over.

A drop of sweat trickled down his chest, between his hair-padded flesh and the plastic wrap of the package he had strapped to himself. He needed his hands free in case he needed to climb, run, or fight off a beggar or thief. Or worse.

Will my family be proud of me? Mom treats me as her darling no matter what I do, and for this she will surely forgive me. But my father - so stern and somber-faced all the time. Will he think me an idiot... a hero?

Down the street Rashid loped like some purposeful ape in a replicated "natural habitat" in a zoo. In a few meters he would be at the fence. Once there, if anyone saw him, they'd know he was up to no good.

I know mom will understand. But Amahl, Samih and my soccer buddies. Will they judge me a fool and laugh at me?

They should be grateful that at least one of us accomplished something. Something which none of them had the courage to do.

The light was dimming, the shadows deepening. *Finally.*

The Barrier

Some distance away, where the traffic could pass, the wall was made of stone and wood. But at Rashid's crossing place it was chain link fencing, secured every two meters by heavy steel posts sunk into concrete pilings. Chunks of the fence bottom had been dragged up from the earth in several spots; in some places by a rodent or a dog, but in others by human hands, to allow the passing of some minor contraband, or perhaps an entire human being with a more substantial package to deliver.

Like mine. This will be taken seriously. This will not be forgotten.

Rashid hauled up on the section he had selected a few days earlier and crawled through the ragged hole in the metal fence.

The illumination at the checkpoint 100 meters to his right would actually help to hide him. The bright lights made it easier for the guards to check the identity papers of the trucks seeking passage. This same brightness made it hard for the guards to see anything in the distance.

As Rashid crawled out from under the fence links he shot a glance towards the checkpoint to assess the risk of discovery. He saw a soldier - a woman. Pale blonde hair and a light-skinned face. So foreign to this part of the world. She was all in khaki, with a large caliber automatic pistol on her waist, a 25-millimeter black leather-handled knife in a sheath strapped to her leg - and that lightweight, fast-firing TAVOR slung over her shoulder.

So long as a random searchlight doesn't hit me, or a military truck doesn't pass by, I should be able to make it. At least to the other side.

Overhead, dim light bulbs barely lit the graying street.

Rashid dashed across like some oversized rat. He darted into a murky spot, what had once been a small alley between two buildings but was now obstructed by a rough-made, waist-high wall. In the darkness, he could crouch low out of the glare of the searchlights or the passing trucks' headlamps.

As he glided into the reassuring darkness, he realized someone was there. Already hiding in the shadow.

Rashid said nothing. *A lover awaiting a clandestine meeting? A husband choosing the right moment to sneak into an illicit tavern? A desperate soul smuggling in some treasure, like German razor blades or American canned peaches in heavy syrup…?* Perhaps it was someone on a mission like his. Rashid said nothing, only listening to the stranger's heavy, determined breathing. Wondering what he would say if challenged. What he would do if a body search was ordered.

The stranger dashed away. Hard-soled footsteps faded quickly into the dark.

Rashid's breath came back to him. He felt along the rough stone wall by his side. This probably had appeared red-brown in the daylight, but by the feeble, naked bulbs above him, the wall was a ghastly, gravestone blue-grey. Choosing a particularly silent moment he stepped out and briskly headed west down the grim street. He knew where he was going. Two streets to go. One more.

As the lights of the university came into view, he unclenched his shoulders a little. He had penetrated far enough into this territory now that he was unlikely to be stopped. In his loose-fitting jeans and bulky brown jacket, he would fit in. He would be just another student heading over to school for an evening class or late session.

Tonight's session will be very special.

The Objective

The campus of Tel-Aviv Peace University / Jerusalem was brightly lit, flaunting its flat green lawns and scrubbed brick walls. In such light no one would see him as a security risk. Rashid stood fully upright.

His warm relief changed to icy apprehension as he considered the steps he'd now need to take to fulfill his mission.

He mounted the steps of the Student Union building with the casual air of a seasoned visitor. As he entered, a neatly-dressed security guard, 50ish and dressed in an ill-fitting uniform the color of grey charcoal with burgundy accents, looked up from his magazine. Following the guard's disinterested nod, Rashid was in.

He thinks he knows me. He thinks we could be friends. Could be friends...

As he entered Meeting Room C, Rashid pasted a calm half-smile on his face to mask his inner anguish. Sharply-dressed students in their twenties, middle-aged professors and older folks were waving at him gently, babbling words of pleasant welcome. He did not let the words' meaning soak in. He would not allow them past his mind's defenses.

He smiled and nodded silently. That was sufficient reply.

They don't know what they've got to look forward to. Many here will find this night difficult to forget.

She was standing near the back of the room: the red-haired Israeli girl. She had returned, and as intriguing as ever. Rashid had desired her from afar, ever since he first came to scout out this location.

This will be the moment. Now, the past ends.

He slowly drew in a deep lungful of air and stepped towards her.

He placed his hands on his chest. The plastic-wrapped surprise under his shirt pressed onto his wet skin.

"Rebeccah, Achdaret Lach Ishi. Ta'ali shufi." (Rebecca, I brought you something. Let me show you.)

Rashid unbuttoned his shirt, grasped the plastic package, undid a flap and extracted the contents which remained dry and intact.

 The Israeli girl's eyes widened in surprise as she saw the package and the bright colors within, turquoise blue and orange.

Rashid continued, "Ta'ala kul attarik min amirika." (I got it all the way from America.)

He passed the garment into her fine, steady hands. She coo-ed with delight as she held it up to the light. Rashid added "Zo Chultza. Memoaadon Hatzchok. Becalifornia?" (It's a T-shirt. From a Laughter Club. In… California?) Rebeccah looked over the shirt silently.

He went on, "Aiwa, da'et'hu kul attarik min amirika." (Yes, I ordered it all the way from America.)

Rebeccah took her eyes away from the package for a moment, and sent her bright blue gaze into Rashid's deep brown eyes - he allowed her gaze to plummet deep into his heart. "Kaneeta lee at zeh behamerica?!" (You got this for me, all the way from America?) she asked.

"Ah, hada min california, alwilayat almutahida." (Yes, it's from California, USA.)

She put the shirt on the table and took Rashid's rough hands into her own. Gazing into his eyes, her smile broadened. Soon she began to giggle.

Rashid began to giggle too.

In three seconds they were laughing, and holding hands, and tossing their heads back. Then they would look in each other's eyes once again, stared at each other for a long second - and burst into laughing and giggling some more.

A lot more.

And thus began a rather memorable evening of the Jerusalem Laughter Club.

-o0o-

Peace - Shalom - Salam

Laughter Mastery

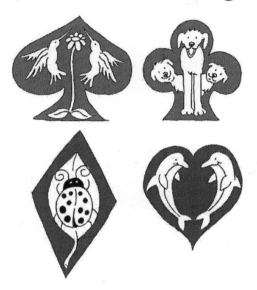

ISBN-13: **978-1979714464**

ISBN-10: **1979714460**

THE LAUGHTER YOGA INSTITUTE

790 Manzanita Drive   Laguna Beach, California   92651 USA
Phone: (949) 376-1939   Cell: (949) 315-5801
Email: info@LYinstitute.org
Web: www.LYinstitute.org

49350480R00098

Made in the USA
San Bernardino, CA
21 August 2019